How to Find Stillness Within

To my teacher, Bernard Bouanchaud, and to T. K. V. Desikachar and his teacher, T. Krishnamacharya

To my love, Miranda, and children, Saffron and Freddie

How to Find Stillness Within

The Yoga Therapy Plan to Help You Find Inner Peace in a Chaotic World

COLIN DUNSMUIR

PENGUIN LIFE

AN IMPRINT OF

PENGUIN BOOKS

PENGUIN LIFE

UK | USA | Canada | Ireland | Australia
India | New Zealand | South Africa

Penguin Life is part of the Penguin Random House group of companies whose addresses can be found at global.penguinrandomhouse.com.

Penguin Random House UK

First published 2022
001

Set in 12/14.75pt Dante MT Std
Typeset by Jouve (UK), Milton Keynes
Printed and bound in Great Britain by Clays Ltd, Elcograf S.p.A.

The authorized representative in the EEA is Penguin Random House Ireland, Morrison Chambers, 32 Nassau Street, Dublin D02 YH68

A CIP catalogue record for this book is available from the British Library

ISBN: 978-0-241-48454-8

www.greenpenguin.co.uk

MIX
Paper from responsible sources
FSC® C018179

Penguin Random House is committed to a sustainable future for our business, our readers and our planet. This book is made from Forest Stewardship Council® certified paper.

Contents

Foreword by Cara Delevingne

Yoga and the *Yoga Sūtra* have completely transformed my life. My teacher, Colin Dunsmuir, introduced me to the wonders and wisdom of this tradition at a time when I was extremely low. I had been battling depression, struggling with work and the trappings and pressures of fame, and feeling completely lost.

With sensitivity and humour, Colin won my trust and I really put him to the test. Most people who know me will tell you I find it very hard to be still, yet he taught me how to be so, and to look inside myself at a time when all I wanted to do was run away. He taught me to sit and breathe and listen; to be quiet when I felt like screaming. He taught me slowly and patiently to move my body with compassion, learning all the while what my biggest obstacles were and how I was getting in the way of myself.

Yoga therapy with Colin was the beginning of what will be a lifelong journey, a continuing process of learning about myself. It has already given me a deep well of understanding that we never have the final answer, but that we can pick up and respond to clues along the way to help prevent ourselves from falling into the same self-sabotaging traps time after time. I have learned that no one and no situation is perfect. I know now that perfection is a myth – each of us has a shadow side and we are all working our way through the circumstances we have been offered, trying to find peace and equilibrium. Colin helped me to find my voice through chanting, and we created rituals I could use as reliable supports to break through my destructive behaviours.

I will be for ever grateful to Colin for bringing me to the wisdom of the ancient yoga texts. I began to immerse myself in their teachings, which I stress-tested over and over and found in their simplicity and depth a cure for my deep depression and self-doubt. I have found an inner resilience that has enabled me to see clearly the harmful patterns I was repeating, and empower me to reject the poor lifestyle choices I had fallen into that had become habitual.

Colin has shown me that yoga is not an exercise, it's a practice. Some days it might feel effortless, on others it will feel like a chore. It's a daily practice that can change shape according to what your body and mind need that day. Trust that yoga will be there for you, and begin to allow it to show you the way. For me, yoga is really about breathwork and meditation. Every time I practise I want to come away having learned something, having grown, having softened, having seen something new about myself or found clarity about a situation that I have been struggling with.

Yoga has above all taught me that we all have to embrace our flaws, that the cracks within us are the beautiful parts that need to have light shone on them. This beautiful and life-affirming book will bring you the deep support and encouragement that I have been so fortunate to have experienced in my life.

Cara Delevingne
London 2022

Introduction

I am one of those smug people who really, truly, loves their job. I find human beings completely fascinating and, as a yoga teacher and therapist, I get to spend my working day talking to people, trying to help them make positive differences in their mind, body and life. I'm constantly impressed by the open-minded curiosity, the agility, passion and humour that people share with me during our conversations. But I'm also witness to their pain, their struggle and confusion. I've been doing this work for more than twenty years now. I've learned that, though we're all different, we're all vulnerable to the same afflictions because that's just part of being human. We get sick. We age. We lose the people we love. We struggle to understand what matters most to us, and what we want to do in the world. Our back aches and our knees creak!

My role as a yoga therapist is to offer people something to relieve their pain: a tool or an insight that will bring real benefit. The tool varies from person to person. It might be a simple set of postures; it could be a mantra. The one constant is to ask lots of questions. I ask questions and then I listen as hard as I can. I encourage the person to listen to their own answers. Even more powerful than a tool to relieve somebody's pain is one that opens their eyes to where that pain comes from.

Conversation isn't necessarily what a new client is expecting from their first session. Those who come to me for yoga therapy are usually looking for relief from a specific problem, whether that's back pain or stress. Those who come to me to deepen their understanding of yoga practice are often looking for new insights or techniques. Either way, they arrive with the expectation that I'll be telling them what to do or passing on new information. They imagine that we'll dive into practising breathing and postures, mantras and meditations. So they're surprised when we just . . . chat. There is a particular look on the faces of some of my new clients, which I spot as our session approaches its close. We've talked for forty-five minutes, maybe more, before I even ask them to try a posture. As we finish, I see them realizing that they've been reflecting on their answers to my questions as they breathed, or stretched, or chanted. They've begun to investigate for themselves where the pain comes from, and are thinking of ways to relieve it.

I love this moment. It's the starting point for a journey into what I refer to as 'True Yoga', which is a voyage of self-discovery. Many people think of yoga first and foremost as a system of exercise, perhaps with some relaxing or calming benefits thrown in. I'm on a mission to show you that there is so much more to it than that. For me, yoga is like an overlooked superpower, hiding in plain sight. It's a form of meditation, a tool for profound self-examination and a means to deepen your relationships with others. It's a system of lived philosophy that has been helping people for thousands of years. It's a spiritual path if you want it to be, but yoga won't force spirituality on you if that's not your thing.

Above all, it's about increasing your understanding of who you really are. Yoga supports us to clarify our perception of the world, of other people and of ourselves. When we see more clearly and know more about our most intimate realities, our yoga practice becomes integrated into our lives. We open our minds to question our reality, our beliefs, our actions and our interactions with others. We practise postures, mantras and breathing to explore further. And then we reflect, via meditation, on what has come up, which brings us back to the questioning. Then the process repeats, moving us in spirals of greater awareness and positivity until every interaction we have, either with our own thoughts or with another person, becomes an opportunity to practise yoga. In this way we are empowered to reduce our unhappiness and struggles and increase our capacity for joyful, purposeful living. Now *that's* yoga. Crow pose? Nice to have but not essential.

I hope that you will join me on a path that takes you deeper and deeper into a clear understanding of how your mind works, where your feelings come from and how to uncover what makes you uniquely *you*. The rewards are greater self-confidence and more resilience, higher energy and much more self-acceptance. This doesn't all happen overnight, of course. The path towards yoga takes years of sustained effort. But it's really, truly, worth it.

Yoga practice vs yoga therapy

Sometimes I think that the wellness industry has eaten yoga and spat it out as a performance for its Instagram followers. I try not to be despondent because I really believe that yoga is such a powerful tool for wellbeing that any and all yoga is good. But I do love to teach people how much more there is for them, lying just beneath the surface.

I teach yoga one-on-one, in the way I learned it from a succession of wonderful teachers. I am privileged to have studied in India, first as a yoga practitioner and then as a yoga therapist, with T. K. V. Desikachar, the son of legendary guru T. Krishnamacharya, and a great teacher and a pioneer of yoga therapy. Krishnamacharya inspired countless other great teachers of modern yoga, including B. K. S. Iyengar, Pattabhi Jois and Indra Devi.

If yoga is a long-term journey into self-knowledge, with huge benefits for general wellbeing, yoga therapy is the application of yoga knowledge to resolve a specific problem. The problem might be felt in the body or mind, the heart or soul, in a person's relationships with others or in their relationship with themselves. Whether it's back pain or stress, a conflicted relationship with a parent or low self-esteem, treatment will require tackling it as an interconnected issue. A yoga therapist is someone who considers people in the round rather than as a cluster of symptoms. All yoga therapists have undertaken long training as yoga practitioners, so they are in a position to direct yoga's powerful tools towards the goal of helping somebody ease their problems.

It's my hope to work with you as I work with my yoga therapy clients, to identify what's troubling you and to begin to apply yoga's powerful tools and insights so that you experience less struggle and more joy.

This brings us back to yoga as a practice rather than a therapy. When we learn more about the practice of yoga we are deepening our awareness of reality. We are shedding illusions and building our resilience to the chaos of life, which can often feel overwhelming. We are learning how to sit down and just *be*. There's a certain amount of faith involved because we're never going to escape the chaos of life completely, no matter how much yoga we practise, but yoga is essentially optimistic because it tells us that change is always possible. In fact, change is *inevitable*, which means that all our discoveries are potentially useful. In the end, yoga is simply a lifelong experiment in better living.

Learning to be yourself

I had a very interesting conversation with a young woman called Fiona a few months ago, in which we shared a moment of empowering realization. She wasn't feeling great about life, or herself. Her mood and energy were low. For some weeks it had been a real struggle to get out of bed in the morning. She was in her final year at school and living at home. Her parents, both of whom I'd worked with in the past, were getting worried about her because when they asked her what was wrong, she simply said, 'I don't know.' So they suggested that we learn together.

Fiona and I talked about her health, her mood, her sleep, her diet, her relationships and her plans. I asked questions and listened as closely as I could to her answers. I invited her to listen to herself, particularly when she was telling me about tension with a certain member of her extended family. We talked about her interactions with that person – their conversations and text messages. How could she change her communication to be clearer, and so dial down her stress?

Our conversation was guided by the wisdom of an ancient text called the *Yoga Sūtra of Patañjali*, usually abbreviated to just the *Yoga Sūtra*, which is the foundation of how I practise my own yoga and how I conduct my yoga therapy work. (It's also the foundation on which this book has been written, so we'll be coming back to it before long.)

We talked through Fiona's responses to some of the *Yoga*

Sūtra's key questions. What makes you feel stable and comfortable? What makes you feel *un*stable and *un*comfortable? It turned out that Fiona was struggling with various relationships, and the only thing that made her feel a bit better was hiding in bed or going out for long walks alone.

I helped her to uncover that she was angry with her relative, and that those feelings were destabilizing her other relationships. We explored the idea that these feelings were not as unacceptable as she believed they were. Perhaps they didn't need to be banished but simply allowed. I suggested that Fiona could and would find a way to tweak her communications so as to produce less anger and more understanding on both sides. Above all, I told her to trust herself.

Towards the end of our discussion, I suggested that she try a simple breathing exercise. She sat in her chair with both feet firmly planted on the ground and with her eyes closed, and I showed her how to slow her breathing and extend her out-breath. It was the first time she'd ever done anything like this but it seemed to help her. She had arrived to our conversation looking tense and withdrawn, but after the ten minutes of gentle breathing, and the grounding awareness of her feet on the floor, she seemed much more relaxed.

And then, as we were wrapping up our chat, I saw it. The look that says, 'I see what triggers my back pain . . . [or my overeating, or my wanting to hide in bed, etc.]. And now that I see it, I feel a bit better. I need to see more clearly and then try to change how I act and react. And that's yoga!' (The way Fiona described it aloud was simply that she'd 'got some perspective'.)

I haven't met with Fiona again, but I hear she's up and about, and back at school and seeing friends. I don't think one yoga session cured her malaise or changed the way she thinks about her life, but I do believe that asking and answering those questions about comfort and stability as honestly as she could gave her a glimpse of a different way to see her reality. It's up to her how far she wants to go down the path towards self-knowledge that we began to explore. I hope she keeps moving towards living at ease with her body, her thoughts and feelings, and with other people. I hope she carries on learning to be herself. I want the same thing for you, too.

My yoga story

I found yoga by accident. Growing up, I'd always been fit and healthy. I worked out and tried to eat well and look after myself. But when I was in my early twenties I developed a stomach ulcer and eventually became so ill I almost died. I had no idea what was wrong with me and ignored the discomfort until one day I collapsed at home. Fortunately, a friend found me, crippled and virtually hallucinating from the pain, and got me to a hospital where they diagnosed a bleeding ulcer in my duodenum. I had to have an emergency operation and was given six pints of blood. The stomach ache I'd been ignoring had nearly killed me.

The operation was a success, but then began the long process of recovery. I had lost a lot of weight and had no energy, but, more than anything, I was shaken. I was a fit young man and I had nearly died. How had it come to this?

I didn't dwell for long on this question. I just wanted to get better. I had always been very driven, very focused with both my fitness and my diet. I was always pushing a bit harder, aiming for more discipline and better results. But I couldn't go back to the gym, at least not for a while. I hired a personal trainer and it was she who suggested yoga as a way slowly to build up my strength. I didn't know anything about yoga except that it was supposed to be gentle, and for the first time in my life, gentle sounded good.

So I went along to try it. I was the only guy in the class. I was *that* guy: the stiff, uncomfortable bloke at the back of the room, feeling out of place. I was either pushing myself too hard (as usual) or barely doing anything because I'd completely missed the point of what I was being shown.

I didn't have an epiphany on my yoga mat that first day, but I did feel a bit better after the class. I went again. And again. Before long I was going three times a week, then four, then five. I was hooked.

Yoga helped me to recover from an acute illness, but it also gave me the opportunity to look at what had made me ill in the first place. It opened my mind to thinking about what made me feel good, or bad, right now. I'd been carrying a whole load of misery and self-doubt around with me for years before I developed the ulcer. Working out had distracted me and allowed me to burn off some of my emotional stress, but the burden never really went away.

Over time, I realized that yoga helped me to feel happier even after the class was over. The more I sat on my mat and paid attention to how a posture made me feel, or to the thoughts that came up when I meditated, the more I started to see things differently. I began to be able to rewrite my story.

My distress was the legacy of an unhappy childhood and adolescence. I had never felt good enough as a child. I was adopted, and I felt my brother was always preferred to me. I used to feel so jealous, so frustrated. I didn't really know where I belonged or who I was. By the time I got sick I had created a detailed and highly polished tale out of these raw materials. The story starred me as the victim, the poor little odd one out who wasn't wanted, loved or valued enough by anybody. Naturally, I was pretty angry about this. Some days I blamed myself, other days I blamed everybody else. And then all that resentment and jealousy and sadness caught up with me. It literally ate away at my insides.

When I started yoga, the initial goal was simply to get fitter. Yoga was one of the only strength-building exercises I could do in my early recovery, and it felt good to be moving my body again, to be gaining flexibility and muscle tone. Then it began to feel good to calm my mind and to connect my mind with my body via my breath. As time went on the rewards kept coming, and they became subtler and more profound.

It wasn't easy. I basically spent the first two years sobbing on my yoga mat. A lot of the time I had no idea what I was crying about. Gradually, I was able to figure it out. Some of my tears were for the little boy I used to be; others were tears of shock and relief that I had come so close to death and survived; others were for the selfish and narcissistic young man I'd become.

I know now that all of this is completely normal. When you begin to practise yoga regularly (or to do any other kind of meditation practice), stuff comes up. Not all of it is pretty and some of it shows you in a bad light. It's best to be prepared for this. That way you can settle in to working with what you discover, rather than getting freaked out.

I had the good fortune to be guided through the process by some incredible teachers, who supported me to re-examine my story of myself and then to rewrite it, so that I was no longer a victim and I no longer needed to blame myself or anyone else. I was helped to see that the story had become the problem, and my illness and recovery provided an opportunity to change it. Yoga has been the central pillar of my life ever since. I have spent nearly twenty-five years refining my own practice, training as a teacher of yoga and, eventually, as a yoga therapist and trainer of yoga therapists.

When I was in my late twenties, my then teacher introduced me to a man called T. K. V. Desikachar (TKV). He was the latest in a long line of yogis stretching back hundreds of years. Like his father, T. Krishnamacharya (TK), he worked hard to make yoga accessible to Westerners. He had enormous experience and insight, built on absolute faith in the tradition of yoga.

Unsurprisingly, he also had a pretty traditional approach to teaching. I very much wanted to study with him, as did lots of other people, but not all of us were ready and motivated to do so, or even to recognize when we were being offered an opportunity to learn. The day I arrived to begin my internship with his organization in India, for example, nearly ended my learning before it had even begun.

I bowled up to the school in Chennai, full of excitement and feeling pretty pleased with both life and myself. I'd been accepted to come by the great man himself. I'd travelled over from the UK and was raring to get started. I presented myself promptly at 9 a.m. at the reception desk in the cramped and stuffy lobby, expecting to be ushered straight through. Instead, I was invited to take a seat. Somebody would come to collect me in due course.

So I took a seat. The overhead fan buzzed with every rotation of its blades. This was back in the days where there was no air con. It got hotter and hotter. I waited until lunchtime and then I told the receptionist I was just popping out for some food. I had a quick lunch, came back and inquired when I might be seen. Soon, I was assured, with a wide and friendly smile. I settled down again to wait.

I was, shall we say, a little surprised when it got to the end of the day and the receptionist (a different one by now) invited me to come back tomorrow. But I told myself that there must have been more pressing issues to deal with that day. No problem.

So I went back the next day. Same thing. By midday I was feeling a bit miffed. After all, I'd come a really long way. Did they know who I was? By the evening, trudging back to my cheap hotel, I was beginning to wonder if they had forgotten I was even coming.

That night I turned it all over in my mind. Was this some kind of joke? No, I realized. Not a joke: a test. A test of how motivated and how ready I was to learn. This was nothing to do with the ego of the master and everything to do with the readiness of the pupil. The question being posed to me, as I sat in that stifling waiting room, was whether I was able to see beyond my wounded ego, my fear of failure, my desire to be special, my identity as the chosen one, my discomfort and lack of ease, and to perceive that I was being offered an opportunity to learn something about myself. Did I have enough healthy motivation to see me through the wait? And was I really ready to be there? My answer to both questions – and I'm so grateful this was the case – was 'yes'.

On the fourth day, at about 11 a.m., a smiling assistant opened a door and gestured to me to follow. No mention was made of the wait. She welcomed me. I thanked her. We began.

I spent years travelling back and forth to India, working with TKV and with various members of his family as well as many other gifted teachers. I learned so much from all of them, but the most important thing I learned was that I didn't need to be Indian, or born into a long line of yogis, or a Hindu or a vegetarian or anything else to practise yoga. All I needed was to be humble, patient, committed and curious enough to use yoga as a tool to find the wisdom already lodged inside me. My current teacher is an exceptional yogi based in France, whom I had to beg for four years to teach me. (There's a theme here!) I spend an hour a day with him, over Zoom. I am still learning.

Yoga therapy is now both my day job and my passion. I support my clients to identify the yoga tools that might help tackle both the symptoms and the root of their problems. Over time, as the person learns through their practice, we modify and add to their personal yoga toolkit.

Profound shifts can arise from this work. Sometimes a person comes for help with IBS and stays to sort out their low self-esteem. Over and over again, I see how yoga heals people. I've practised yoga therapy in care homes and hospital wards, with patients recovering from acute illness and those who are end-of-life. Yoga can comfort a dying person's heart even as their body is shutting down. It can soothe a wounded mind. It can heal our very sense of who we are.

How to use this book

It doesn't matter whether you're a beginner or an experienced yogi because this book is emphatically not a programme to follow week by week or month by month. It won't teach you postures and it won't assume any prior knowledge. Whether you're a dabbler or a devotee doesn't matter to me. I don't care whether you're doing Haṭha, Iyengar, Vinyāsa or any other kind of physical practice. In fact, for the purpose of this book it really doesn't matter whether you've ever set foot in a yoga class at all.

All that matters is that you are curious enough about yoga to investigate it from a different angle: not as a sequence of moves but as a mindset. That mindset was described brilliantly more than 2,000 years ago in a collection of verses, or *sūtra*, called the *Yoga Sūtra*, attributed to a mysterious individual known as Patañjali. He (or she?) was not so much the author as a channel for collective wisdom. After being handed down for many generations from teacher to student using oral tradition, the *Yoga Sūtra* was eventually written down, in Sanskrit, by scholars in India some 500 years ago. It has become a foundation of modern yoga and will be our guide throughout this book.

The book is shaped by one of many possible journeys through the text of the *Yoga Sūtra*, one that I've used many times with different clients. We're not going to start at the beginning and carry on until we get to the end. We'll be focusing on chapters one and two (out of four), which set out some of the fundamentals of yoga as both philosophy and practice, and nipping around from one group of lines to another, mining them for insights that we can use in everyday life. In this way we'll be learning how to practise yoga in a way that unleashes its power and makes it personal for us. Not so much standard sequences of postures as nuggets of wisdom that you can string together in endlessly different and beautiful ways, according to your needs.

If this sounds challenging, please don't worry. There will be plenty of guidance and lots of real-life stories along the way. Yoga isn't complex in its essence. It is simply another word for 'meditation'. It allows you to bring gentle but steady awareness to your present moment and, in that way, make discoveries about yourself and the world. It is this awareness that enables you to change, whether that's reacting differently to a relative who presses your buttons or choosing healthy ways to relax rather than always reaching for a glass of wine.

As you gain experience, your trust in your intuition grows. You will begin to experience a virtuous circle in which your confidence flourishes as you see positive results, and you get better results as you learn to find the exercises, mantras or insights you need on any given day. This intuitive and experimental approach explains why the book is organized around different sections in the *Yoga Sūtra* rather than, for example, a week-by-week programme.

In Chapter 1 I explore yoga in terms of what it can offer us and how to approach it: as a way of life rather than a life hack. I also introduce you to the wisdom of the *Yoga Sūtra*. I explain a little about what it is and how it sustains my practice and teaching. Most important of all, I set out how it can be your personal guide on your own exploration of yoga.

Chapters 2 to 4, which guide you through the text of the *Yoga Sūtra*, are divided into sections or 'groups' exploring a line's possible meaning in our contemporary world. In these three chapters you will notice a series of questions appearing at the end of the chapter, inviting you to review what you have read and assimilate it into your own experience. Asking questions and paying attention to the answers is at the heart of what I do, and what I help my clients to do. I hope that you will be able to use these questions to build your understanding of your mind and behaviours at the same time as you learn more about yoga. I always encourage people to deepen their awareness of their thoughts and emotions as a first step, and only then experiment with different postures, mantras and breathing exercises. It's so important to prepare our minds and deepen our understanding of what yoga is, and what it is not. Otherwise, we take all our misunderstandings straight into our practice. (This is why I don't introduce any exercises until midway through these chapters.)

Then, in Chapter 5, I explore some of the many directions you could take your yoga in if you want to make it into a lifelong practice. Depending on your values and beliefs, that could mean exploring the spirituality of yoga or using it as a deep self-care system that supports you to do activist work.

My deepest wish is that you will find in this book a thread to connect you to the wisdom contained in the *Yoga Sūtra*, but reading it will not make any difference to you unless you also do some work actively in daily life. Yoga is fundamentally dynamic. It's something that you *do* and which brings about change. One of the many ways to define it is as a form of lived philosophy, one that you practise rather than study. So you can't do yoga by reading about it (even in this book!), only by practising it.

That said, it's a big subject and, as with any system, it helps to know how it works and how you can apply it. The aim of this book is to give you enough understanding of yoga to begin to put in place your own practice and to seek out the teachers you need to take that practice deeper. When you approach this task with joyful curiosity, I promise you great things can and will happen. You will be able to replace unhealthy habits with healthier ones, move on from toxic relationships and experience more relaxation, joy and purpose.

There is no correct or incorrect place from which to begin your yoga practice. For most of us, the starting point is a group class focused on postures. That's how it was for me. But it could just as well be a meditation practice, or a breathing exercise. It could be a YouTube video or an Instagram story. All of these routes are valid.

Yoga really is a process of trial and error, of figuring out what helps and what doesn't. It can never be prescriptive because we are all different from one another. In fact, endless variety and difference are even more prevalent than that, because we're not just different from one another but different *from ourselves, day by day*. As T. K. V. Desikachar said in his book *The Heart of Yoga*, every student of yoga is a different person today from the person they were yesterday. Yoga must be flexible enough to treat each of us anew every time we show up.

Please view this book as a signpost on your journey, not as a manual. There is no right or wrong way to do yoga. I meant it when I said that it doesn't matter what kind of physical practice you're doing, or not doing. The one thing I really passionately care about is that you grasp how much more there is to yoga than the postures. It contains a whole universe of tried and trusted ways to bring comfort and stability into every aspect of your life. And with that in place, it can be a gateway to deep joy and calm contentment, to passionate and compassionate and purposeful living. I hope you enjoy exploring.

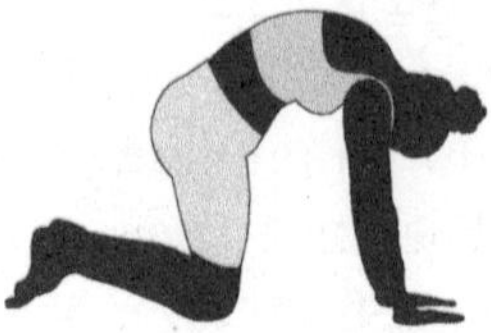

1. *Yoga as Way of Life*

You could be forgiven for thinking that you already know what yoga is. If you practise it yourself, then (hopefully) you know that it can relax or energize you, calm the nerves, stretch away muscle tension and build core strength. Even if you don't, you probably have a sense of what yoga involves, and that it's somehow 'good for you'. After all, in its physical aspect – the postures that most of us think of if someone says 'yoga' – it is very visible in our wellness-obsessed culture. Yoga is all over Instagram and YouTube. There are daily classes at local leisure centres and in studios up and down the land.

It is brilliant that so many people are already benefiting from their yoga practice. Whether they use it to combat insomnia or back pain, deal with injury, or for stretching and relaxation, it's wonderful that millions of us have yoga in our lives. But there's so much more to it than what we see from the back of a crowded class once a week. I'm on a mission to open people's eyes to what yoga can enable them to do. And I'm not talking about holding advanced postures for twenty minutes straight.

Yoga is the most profound system of self-care I've ever come across because it's founded on self-knowledge. It shows you how to integrate every aspect of yourself, and in the process discover your purpose. And the best thing is that, for all its profundity, it's also remarkably simple. Yoga teaches us to start from where we are, beginning with the breath. There are no other requirements. As T. Krishnamacharya said, 'If you can breathe, you can do yoga!' I still get excited about this amazing truth: that when breath and body and mind are brought together in conscious awareness, great changes occur. If this resonates with you, that's wonderful – and welcome aboard!

Introducing the Yoga Sūtra

Aside from realizing that anyone can be a yogi so long as they have the right attitude, the crucial takeaway from my time in India was my discovery of the *Yoga Sūtra*, which is more a manual for how to do life than a guide to postures or instructions on how to breathe or meditate. It is a detailed exploration of the mindset that you move into when you practise yoga, as well as how to evolve and change.

I studied the *Yoga Sūtra* the old-fashioned way, not by reading but by listening, repeating and memorizing it. My fellow students and I had to repeat what our teacher chanted, verse by verse. As we progressed through the *sūtra*, we would be given an example drawn from everyday life to show us exactly what each line meant. More than the literal meaning of the words, we needed a practical understanding of what each *sūtra* signified. The real test of understanding came when the teacher asked us to give an example from our own life of the idea contained in the *sūtra*. We would repeat this process of listening, chanting, telling stories and sense-checking as many times as it took to satisfy our teacher that we had truly incorporated the *sūtra* into our whole being.

As a method of learning, this oral tradition felt positively medieval. (Actually, it was even older – this is how teachers and pupils studied all over the ancient world, and in every culture where there was no written language.) But though it was archaic, it was also highly effective. I loved that it was so deeply practical. We weren't just memorizing words, or even focusing on the poetry of the Sanskrit language. We learned the significance of those words by bringing the *sūtra* into our own everyday lives.

Yoga can, of course, be practised in a way that emphasizes its mystical or esoteric side, and I see the appeal of this approach, but to my mind, the reason for yoga's incredible effectiveness is precisely its insistence that we envelop the esoteric within the everyday. This is what so impressed and moved me when I was studying in Chennai. I hope to be able to pass on just a little of that sense of excitement and possibility through this book.

The *Yoga Sūtra* is an incredible blend of psychology and philosophy. If that makes it sound a bit heavy, I should say that it's pretty short, only 195 lines. And beneath the poetic language, its message is simple: positive change is achievable for all of us. If you pay close attention to what you do, think and feel, you can refine your actions in order to suffer less. From there, your life is yours for the exploring!

It is a manifesto that describes how to wake up to life's possibilities and awaken your own. For me and countless others, it has been transformational. I love the fact that it still feels so relevant, even though it was written in such a different culture and context from our own. Despite that gulf of difference, it can still guide us to make practical changes in our lives. It feels universal. I never tire of applying a line of wisdom from the *Yoga Sūtra* to help someone get a grip on their addiction to social media, say, or dial down the conflict with their partner, or manage their anxiety over parenting.

The text frequently discusses the blockages on our paths through life, and how they are always the product of our own minds. They develop from things like our fears and desires and our egos. It is constantly nudging us to ask questions about what's getting in our way and where it's come from. How have old feelings been processed, via our memories and through the power of our imaginations, into stories? Do those stories serve us? What do we believe about ourselves and the world? What are we attached to? What are we *over*-attached to? What do we identify with? *How* do we identify? Why? These are the questions that shape my work and that will shape this book and your journey through it.

I want to tell you a brief story to show you what I mean. I've been talking to a woman called Kelly for a number of years now. During the time we've known each other she's become a mother and moved out of London to live in the countryside with her husband and daughter. There are lots of things about this move that she loves, but feeling cut off from family and friends as she struggles with how to parent her three-year-old is not one of them. Kelly has a tight-knit group of people she trusts but she struggles to make new friends. She's always had the belief that she's an introvert who doesn't get on with people. In addition, she grew up feeling like the odd girl out in her group, most of whose families were wealthier than hers.

So now she's living in a village, taking her daughter to playgroup and music sessions in the village hall and trying to make friends for herself but also, crucially, for her child. And life is feeling harder and harder.

A few months ago, Kelly became very distressed over her relationship with her daughter, who was having a lot of tantrums. They were always fighting. I asked her what they fought about. 'Just the normal clash of wills you get with a toddler,' she said. Tantrums can feel really challenging, I know, but on its own, this didn't seem like reason enough to be fighting so much.

Eventually, Kelly told me she no longer wanted to go out to their various activities, in case there was 'a scene'. But she didn't want to invite people round for play dates either because her house was so much smaller than all the other mothers' houses. The one time she had invited a little boy and his mum over, she had been very anxious, tidying up for hours beforehand and then gritting her teeth all the way through, dreading that the other mum wouldn't enjoy herself, or that the food she had provided for the children was wrong, or that her daughter would have a tantrum and she would be unable to manage it appropriately. She decided that there would be no more play dates.

So Kelly and her child were getting more and more isolated. She felt she was letting her daughter down. Their relationship was getting worse and poor Kelly told me she felt like a complete failure. Why wasn't it easy? She loved her daughter and loved being a mum. She had her husband for support. She had a lovely cottage, a garden, the peace and tranquillity she had craved when she was living in London. She talked to her mum every day on Zoom. But none of it was helping her to feel stable and comfortable.

We spent some time digging into why she didn't want to have people over. We followed the threads of her painful childhood memories and also looked at the way she was projecting those memories into her child's future. We looked at the way her belief that she was an introvert, and so couldn't be expected to manage social interactions, was in tension with her belief that she was a good mother who put her child's needs first. We did a lot of talking.

Since we know each other well, we trust each other enough to be completely honest. I suggested to her that when beliefs about our identity clash in a painful way, it's an opportunity to have another look at them. Was she really socially awkward and shy? Or was she simply a person who was still scared of the judgement of her peers? There was one fellow mother she instinctively liked and trusted more than any of the others. This woman had already demonstrated that she was an ally, showing understanding when Kelly's daughter had had a melt-down in the playground. What about if she invited her over?

Eventually, Kelly agreed that this was a risk worth taking. I challenged her to set a time limit on how long she would tidy up for beforehand, and to stick to it. We ran through the breathing exercises she could use to anchor herself in the present moment and calm her anxiety. And I referred her back to some lines of the *Yoga Sūtra*. (E.g. How could she do something differently?)

An important thing to know about Kelly is that she takes everything away from our sessions, does her practice, reflects again and incorporates what she learns into her life. And repeat. In other words, she does the work. So what comes next in this story should be understood in that context. It wasn't anything I said to her that led to a successful outcome, it was the work she put in.

Anyway, Kelly agreed to that play date and it went fine. Better than fine. So I suggested something even braver. What about if she decided to invite several people over? Two or three kids at a time, complete with parents. A little party. What if she filled her house with people?

Because she'd already had some success, she agreed. We ran through all the meditation and posture work she would practise every day: twenty minutes in the morning and twenty minutes at bedtime, to support her new trial approach. And the following week she told me that she and her daughter had had a great week. They hadn't fought once. And she'd even enjoyed the sight of her house full of people, which challenged her belief that social interaction was painful for her.

She told me that she'd been able to bring her attention back to the lines in the *Yoga Sūtra* about the futility of our deep need to know and understand what's happening around us. This inability to be comfortable with *not knowing* is at the heart of all other lack of comfort. It can lead to a sense that we aren't strong enough to cope with a situation. We don't know what to do when our child is lying screaming on the floor. We don't know what someone thinks of the way we respond. We never really know what to do for the best, how to interpret the past or plan for the future. We are overwhelmed by this not knowing and we get controlling, angry or afraid.

The *Yoga Sūtra* says that our inability to tolerate not knowing is the root of all our struggles in life. It comes along with fear, attachment, aversion and desire. We can't just let things be, see what happens and trust we will be agile enough to respond in the moment. Feeling fearful, we hold on tight to our plans or beliefs about how things must be. But the tighter we grip, the more we wobble and the more we suffer.

Kelly told me that she came back to this thought many times during the group play date. She visualized the words and encouraged herself to settle more comfortably into not knowing whether a tantrum was on the way, or how everyone would behave if it was. She encouraged herself to be OK with that. And it helped. She suffered less, both at the time and afterwards. That act of paying attention in the moment, combined with careful preparation beforehand and reflection afterwards, was enough to tip Kelly out of a vicious cycle and into a more positive one. She's not 'cured'. She's just a little more comfortable and a little more stable, with a bit more energy to keep walking the path she's on.

One definition of the Sanskrit word *sūtra* is 'verse', as in verses or lines in a poem. Another (more literal) definition is 'thread'. Many yoga scholars discuss the *Yoga Sūtra* as a collection of threads, woven together to make an intricate whole. For me, an even more beautiful metaphor is to think of these *sūtra* unspooling like a rope of wisdom, left for us by our ancestors to guide us through life. In Greek mythology, Theseus unrolled a ball of thread as he made his way through the labyrinth, looking for the Minotaur. It was such a complex maze that if he hadn't left this thread to guide him on the way out, he would have been trapped inside for ever. Life can seem like a labyrinth. I feel lucky to have found this thread that guides and connects me to all the people who've made their way before me. I hope that the *Yoga Sūtra* will be a guiding thread for you, too.

Yoga for real people in a real world

Yoga holds no meaning when it's only a theory. There is no such thing as the one 'true' yoga; there is only yoga in practice. When we practise yoga, we discover for ourselves what yoga is. So what follows is simply an outline of the basics of how I understand it. I hope they act as pointers to set you on your way.

As I'm sure you've grasped by now, there's much more to discover in yoga than *āsana* (pronounced *ah*-sana) or postures. In terms of the tools of yoga practice, there are many other elements that don't get nearly as much airtime in yoga classes, such as breathwork, voicework via mantras, and visualization.

And as we've been seeing, the purpose and promise of yoga, and the reason for using all these tools, is not so much to get into impressively bendy postures as to gain more understanding of our emotions, our decision-making and the way we interact with people. So that's my first point about what yoga *isn't*. It's not (just) about the headstands.

What is it, then? I believe that yoga is a tool for paying attention. When we practise yoga we are linking the essence of ourselves, via our attention, with an object. That object could be anything – a thought or a person or an activity. We will come back to look more closely at the essence of ourselves, as well as these objects, later on. For now, it's the quality of the attention (calm, detached enough to consider an object from different angles, enveloping and gentle) that I want to use to define yoga. Most simply, yoga is meditation.

But it's not just about the quality of what's going on inside your mind, crucial though that is. The reason we aim for this quality of meditative mind is so that we can understand reality more clearly. The first object of our meditation is our relationship with our selves. Yoga is a means for creating more harmonious connections between all the different elements of our being: body, mind, heart and soul. For example, it teaches us to detach from our thoughts enough to realize that they are not us. Gradually, we learn to bring awareness to many of our internal objects, from noticing the inner voices we use to talk to ourselves to seeing that how we nourish our bodies (or not) affects our minds. Yoga allows us to explore the ecosystem that is our being.

Yoga has a lot to offer in the world of social and emotional and personal interactions, too. Once you've begun to bring more awareness to your relationship with yourself, you're well placed to use yoga to gain insight into the dynamics of your relationships with other people, from friends and family to co-workers and romantic partners. So yoga is also a system for improving relationships.

Ultimately, yoga shows you how to be more *you*. It is the road map to more authentic, peaceful, joyful and purposeful living. It poses the question, 'Who am I, really?' and gives us a way to find out. Yoga shows us the possibility of who we *could* be.

In yoga, your lived experience is valid and meaningful. The reality you experience is your best guide to creating change that works for you. You do not need to follow what a guru says, or live by the rules of a sacred text. You are your own centre of wisdom. That said, it is the opposite of ego-bound self-indulgence. Yoga is not 'me time'. It encourages you to make positive change in your own being so that you can bring about positive change in the world. So, while it puts you at its centre, yoga is not all about you.

And while we're on the subject of gurus and sacred texts, yoga is a philosophy, not a religion. It grew out of the rich mystical tradition that has also given the world Hinduism, but yoga is not a branch of Hinduism. The *Yoga Sūtra* can be viewed by Hindus as a religious text, but nowhere does it present itself in those exclusive terms. Yoga, as it is currently practised all over the world, including in India, is non-dogmatic, non-ideological and completely compatible with any religious, spiritual or philosophical beliefs you already hold. It doesn't require you to believe in anything or anyone, only to observe yourself and others closely and to take action to bring about beneficial change.

Given this, it's no surprise that yoga has no entry requirements. Yoga doesn't care how old you are, or how young. You can be eighty or eighteen and still benefit. You don't have to be skinny, or super fit or bendy, or into wellness to do yoga. You don't have to be vegan. There's no ideal body type for yoga. All you need is a sense of curiosity and some patience. And both of these can be developed so long as you approach your practice with an open mind, ready and willing to learn.

My next point is a (sort of) warning. I have to be straight with you: yoga is not a life hack. It rewards people who adopt the 'small-actions-taken-often' approach to change, rather than those who prefer a burst of intense activity once in a while. It's really not a quick fix, and if you want to see long-lasting change, prepare yourself for the fact that it could take years.

But though yoga is a challenge, it should not be a struggle. It needs to fit into your life and it needs to work for you. I believe that yoga can help us right from day one, even if it takes years to unpick the big knots of who we are. If you can commit to twenty minutes of yoga practice a day, you're all set. By the end of this book, I hope you will be doing ten minutes in the morning and ten minutes in the evening. This is a fantastic foundation. Yoga, like everything in life, involves a lot of trial and error. It's a great experiment, conducted by you. So go with the ebb and flow of your life and remember, the longer you practise, the deeper your self-knowledge and the more rewarding the results.

Finally, if headstands are not your thing, you're in the right place! Yoga works on many levels and can lead to an infinite variety of changes. It can ease back pain and help to mend a broken heart. It can calm anxiety symptoms, give you perspective on problems and support you through times of stressful change, such as bereavement, a divorce or your children leaving home. It can take you deep into a relationship with a higher being. It can also, if you wish, lead to seriously impressive headstands!

2. *Laying the Foundations*

Welcome to your exploration of yoga. This is the first of three chapters that cover a route through the first two chapters of the *Yoga Sūtra*. Chapter One defines yoga and describes the mindset that is the foundation of yoga practice. Chapter Two gives more detail on how we can attain that mindset. (Chapter Three explores meditation themes in a more detailed and esoteric way and Chapter Four offers a sort of treatise on yoga for leaders, activists and people working with responsibility for others. Both are fantastically insightful and rewarding, but they're a bit 'next level' for my purposes in this book.)

We will be focusing in this chapter on preparing to practise yoga by deepening your awareness of what your mind gets up to and why. This awareness of mind, of its activities and the obstacles that get in its way, is the foundation of yoga.

As we've seen, yoga is fundamentally a system for understanding ourselves and our interactions with the world. It's psychology as well as philosophy, and the *Yoga Sūtra* reflects that. Unlike many other ancient Indian texts, it doesn't use parables about gods or goddesses to convey its wisdom. It's written as an investigation of what it is possible to experience with the human mind. It offers tools and techniques to clarify perception, relieve discomfort of every kind and foster a stable mind and a healthy and secure body.

Throughout this chapter and the next two, I will be guiding you on a journey that I've taken many times when teaching yoga therapists or working with clients. It's not a straight path from start to finish of the text. It jumps around all over the place, moving from one group of lines to another. It gives you a route (one among many) through the *Sūtra*'s wisdom and shows you how to incorporate it into your own life. We end back where we started, with a reminder that you could return to the *Yoga Sūtra* throughout your life, reading in different sequences, and find something new every time.

Each group of lines has a theme to prime your exploration. Then, I've tried to sum up the spirit of each line and sometimes used stories to explore it. I've also included the line reference so that you can flip to the complete word-for-word translation at the back of this book if you wish.

Group 1: What are you aiming for?

Comfort + stability = your new life goal (2.46)

We're plunging right into the middle of the second chapter of the *Yoga Sūtra* and a kernel of absolutely golden insight. This line offers a simple vision of yoga in practice. When we are in a state of yoga, it says, we are both comfortable and stable. We see clearly, without misreading situations. We're calm and ready to act in the world. For me, this is a fantastic starting point because it shows us what we're aiming for: to be comfortable and stable both in body and, as our practice deepens, in mind. The two things are totally interconnected, right from the start.

This line also sums up yoga's practical approach. The fundamental question I ask everyone I work with derives from this *sūtra*. What makes you comfortable? What makes you *un*comfortable? What makes you feel stable, or unstable? In other words, what helps and what harms? When we're beginning yoga, it really helps to come back to these questions, over and over again. They seem simple, but their implications are profound.

So what does it mean to be comfortable? I'm not thinking merely about the absence of pain or having the basics of a comfortable life. I'm thinking of comfort that comes from somewhere inside. We might say of somebody, 'He seems really comfortable with himself.' This is a positive quality, implying that somebody knows who he is and values himself, without having to boast about it. It suggests self-awareness and authenticity, an ego that's taking up just the right amount of space. It suggests ease and purpose and warmth. These are the kinds of qualities I associate with feeling comfortable.

How about stability? I used to think that meant strength, a lack of vulnerability to shock, having enough padding, whether through muscle or money in the bank, to guarantee that we (meaning I!) wouldn't get knocked sideways in any sense. Now I think it's more to do with having both feet on the ground. With having points of reference you can trust. If we rely on external points of reference to keep us feeling stable (those muscles, or our bank balance, our marriage or friendship or job title) we're laying ourselves open to terrible instability if any of them change. And change, as I'm sure you know, is inevitable in this life. If we can find our points of reference inside ourselves, we're less likely to topple when that change comes. Our behaviours are likely to be more stable, more familiar to us, more in line with what we know of ourselves.

How do the two states – comfort and stability – complement or interact with one another? For me, being comfortable with yourself is the ultimate stability. By the way, don't forget that what makes you stable at one point in your life might not be what keeps you stable later. 'Stable' is very different from 'rigid'.

Here's the first of your questions for self-reflection. It's the one I've already mentioned, the one I return to time and again in my work . . . We'll be coming back to the concepts of stability and comfort many times, but for now, let's move on.

What makes you comfortable? What makes you uncomfortable? What makes you stable? What makes you unstable?

Use your body and breath to explore your mind (2.47)

In yoga, it really helps to see everything that happens as an opportunity to practise. Every action, every interaction with someone else, is an opportunity to learn about yourself, them, the world. The way you learn is through paying calm and curious attention to your body, your breath and your thoughts and feelings.

So, for example, using your body to explore yoga postures will allow you to notice how much effort you need to make to move into a certain position. Do you need to put more effort in, or perhaps do less? How much effort is just right for it to feel comfortable and stable to you? Can you let go of your own rule that says your hand must be parallel to your foot, if that increases both your comfort and your stability? A rule is only ever a framework, after all. The real learning happens not by following rules slavishly but by learning how to adapt to them and with them.

You don't have to be a master straight away. Simply bringing attention to your breath and body as you sit, walk, do postures or meditate is the perfect way to begin. Gradually you will grow accustomed to slipping into a state of relaxed alertness. You'll get more comfortable with observing your thoughts and feelings, perhaps at first in hindsight but, increasingly, in real time. You'll be able to assess how you respond to criticism, to compliments, to intimacy or someone being distant. You'll begin to intuit ways to get out of painful situations with ease.

In the meantime, of course, shit will happen. At the risk of being irritating, I have to say that even the shit is an opportunity to practise. The next time you get into a row with someone you love, for example, try reminding yourself that, although this situation may be challenging and unpleasant, it's also an opportunity for you to practise not giving your power away. Or not to overreact, or storm off in a huff. This is hard. Patience is key to developing the ability to remain calm and curious about what's going on around you. You can't rush it.

Think back over the last twenty-four hours. Can you identify an opportunity to practise what came up for you? How might you have refined your effort? How could you have adapted? How will you do it differently next time? How could you find the potential to succeed in the long run?

Greater clarity is what it's all about (2.48)

I ask myself, 'What's really going on here?' dozens of times a day. I own a horse and absolutely love riding. My horse and I go out most days. Every single time, I learn something about myself. I had an accident a few months ago, got thrown off and hurt my back. (That wasn't very good for my identity as a yogi, by the way. I was pretty attached to the idea of myself as stable, intuitive and agile. The horse had other ideas and helped to show me a different perspective!)

Ever since, I've worked hard to process my nervousness about being unseated again. I've done a lot of practice to allow that fear to flow through me and now my mind feels clear. But one day a few weeks ago when we were out, I noticed that, although my mind was calm, my body felt tense. The horse was getting tense, too. I asked myself, 'What's really going on here?' and realized that there was fear stuck somewhere within my body and the horse could feel it. I had to give up on riding that day and go home and practise. For me, the question 'What's really going on here?' is the call to see more clearly, to read the reality of the situation I find myself in rather than the projection of what I want it to be. Here, asking the question enabled me to shift from, 'Nothing to see here, I've totally conquered my fear!' to, 'Ah! My mind may be over it, but my body isn't yet.'

With practice, most situations can be viewed with improved clarity. In situations where fear or desire or ego is involved, it is harder to see reality. Relationships, which often involve a potent mix of anxieties and desires and needs and roles, are a breeding ground for difficulties, but every difficulty can be used as an opportunity.

One lady I work with is locked in a roller coaster of

emotions with somebody whom she supports financially yet who is unable to commit to being with her. She's got so used to the drama that she now mistakes it for stability, even if it makes her uncomfortable. She's enabling him to behave in a certain way, and he's refusing to accept her for what she is and what she wants. A little more clarity would be so helpful, but, of course, there's so much fear, desire, ego and attachment going on that it's really hard to achieve.

Calm and curious detachment leads to greater clarity, but it takes practice, and there's always more to learn, as my horse teaches me virtually every day. Yoga continues to teach me, too. 'What's really going on here?' I ask myself as I do my *āsana* practice and feel a twinge. 'Do I need to do more? Or do less?' I ask questions, and experiment and adjust.

The body is our vehicle in life and it expresses what is happening in our minds and with our emotions. It is a tool for self-exploration. *Āsana* with breathing is an embodied experience. When you move into a posture, you're acting out your attitudes, conflicts, needs and relationships, right there on your yoga mat. Do you push hard or do you freak out at the first hint of discomfort? Do you compete with others? Do you strive for perfection? Do you want recognition from the teacher, or reassurance? Every *āsana* is an opportunity to develop greater clarity and to deal gracefully with what you're being presented with, no matter the ups and downs.

> *Tomorrow, when something makes you feel uncomfortable, however small or vague the feeling, ask yourself, 'How will I navigate this?' 'What's really going on here?' 'How can I deal with everyday life successfully?'*

Group 2: What's getting in your way?

So, you're steering a course towards greater comfort and stability. What's blocking you? And what story are you telling yourself that's solidifying these blockages?

Obstacles look at first sight as if they come in all shapes and sizes, and, of course, on one level that's true: every problem is slightly different because so is every person and situation. Some clients tell me that their big block is criticism from an overbearing parent. Others that it's stress from the impossible workload in the office, over-reliance on a partner, daily drinking to numb their feelings, or any number of things that leave them upset, uncomfortable, wobbly and unstable. But while it's clearly true that no individual's life is exactly like anyone else's, our difficulties and responses to difficulty are all driven by the same root causes.

In this group of lines, the *Yoga Sūtra* lists the five roots of all those blocks to our comfort and stability, and shows us that they lie within the mind. So, the problem isn't work stress, for example, it's our terror of slipping up and fear of speaking out about the impossibility of the workload. This is good news because it means that our problems have their origins in our minds, and are therefore ours to tackle.

Difficulties are inevitable, but they don't have to define us (2.3)

In this line, the *Yoga Sūtra* shows us that there are five essential and universal aspects of human nature that sprout like seeds within us and can, if we don't deal with them, grow into serious problems. They are:

- not-knowing (or being unaware),
- ego (or confused references / identity / values),
- desire (or excessive attachment),
- aversion (or judgement),
- fear.

These are known as *kleśa* (pronounced *clay*-sha) and they are both the roots of and the routes to all our difficulties and discomforts.

It's important to realize that they themselves are not the problem. It's not fear that's your issue, for example – it's what you do with fear. Do you deny or evade it, in which case it might eventually manifest as an anxiety disorder or depression, or do you recognize and own it, in which case you might channel it into daring or creativity? Looking at the issue the other way, this line suggests that, instead of seeking a cure for anxiety disorder, we try to understand how the five variables of the *kleśa* are contributing to it and begin to work with them.

Everybody struggles with the *kleśa* and their manifestations to a greater or lesser degree. There is no way we can eliminate them, because they're part of being human and are useful to us, though yoga practice shows us how to reduce their negative impact in our lives.

We'll go on to look at each one in turn, but for now, I also want to emphasize that the *kleśa* generate not merely problems to be solved but also opportunities to learn. This is because, as the *Yoga Sūtra* tells us, they have the potential to be manifested as accompaniments to either negative or positive events in our lives. It all depends what we do with them when they come up.

This is a really challenging idea so I'm not expecting you to absorb it straight away, much less be able to act on it. For now, it's enough to contemplate the suggestion that our problems are not immovable rocks dumped in our path. We can work with the fruits of our confusion, our ego, our desires, fears and aversions. They are more malleable than we perhaps realize and they absolutely do not need to define us.

Can you think of a problem in your own life that felt like an obstacle at the time but now looks more like an opportunity to change something? Can you identify the possible involvement of not-knowing, ego, desire, aversion or fear? Was one primarily in play or several? How did they get in your way? How could you have approached it differently?

The root of our trouble is that we can't see clearly (2.4–2.5)

Not-knowing is the root *kleśa* from which the others grow. Many of us do not really know ourselves, let alone other people. We can't know what's going to happen in the future, or why something happened in the past. We can guess, we can speculate and try to figure it out, but not knowing is the default condition of being alive. There are so many layers of misunderstanding within this general condition of not knowing. We misattribute motivation to others and are blind to our own biases and blocks.

Why is it such a struggle to see reality as it truly is? Because we're all subject both to past conditioning and to the lure of a fantasy life. We're swayed by painful memory or by the temptation to imagine a different life in the future. We project an image of ourselves or we buy into the image that others are projecting. There's a mismatch between what we want reality to be and how it actually is, right here and now.

This can lead to other problems, for example over-attachment or anxiety. We might end up desperate to stay in a romantic relationship with someone who wants to move on. Or we feel too frightened to go out and make new friends because of painful memories of previous rejection by a peer group. In both cases, the desire and the fear are products of misunderstanding. We have misread a situation, failed to perceive it as it actually is, right now in the present, distinct from our ego's needs, desires and fears.

Some people cherish the hope that if they practise yoga for long enough they will transcend misunderstanding. This is completely unrealistic and is driven by ego. In fact, it's a misunderstanding of reality and a projection of our desire to be perfect. So let's get one thing clear: we all get the wrong end of the stick sometimes. That's fine. We're all human.

Rather than try to eradicate not-knowing by knowing more, a better way to work with it is to acknowledge what it is that you don't know. Many of us are terrified of saying, 'I don't know' when we're asked a question, for example. We imagine it makes us look weak, or that we've failed to do our homework. Actually, blustering and posturing make us weak. It is empowering to say, 'I don't know,' if that's the case. It communicates that you're comfortable with yourself, and that builds trust. You learn to trust that you can say this. Other people learn to trust that you don't deal in bullshit. Greater comfort and stability all round . . .

One of the phrases I use most frequently in my work is, 'We need to get more comfortable with not knowing.' I say it a lot, precisely because most of us are so *un*comfortable with not knowing, which means we never settle into it for long enough to spot the opportunities it contains. Try saying 'I don't know' to others and to yourself. With practice, out of your fog of not-knowing will emerge potentially useful insights.

What comes up for you when you sit and just be? You don't have to call this meditation, by the way. It might be when you're on the bus or in the shower. The next time your mind is at rest, try to identify the qualities of what comes up. What emotions do you feel? You don't have to do anything with the feelings or thoughts. Just sit as comfortably as you can with not knowing.

Ego rides to the rescue – and makes everything worse (2.6)

Being confused is uncomfortable (at least until we've learned to embrace it). We prefer to tell ourselves that we know what's going on in our lives; that we've got a plan and are making progress. We tell stories to explain the world and ourselves. All of this planning and storytelling is the product of our egos, which comprise confused values, misperceptions and mistaken beliefs, overreactions, grudges and fantasies. When your ego is working overtime to sort out a mess, you're only sinking deeper into quicksand.

Often, we don't even see that's what's happening because most of us are so overidentified with our egos. It is hard to grasp that there is a difference between the conscious part of ourselves, doing the perceiving, and the thoughts or feelings that are being perceived. Most of us assume that our thoughts and feelings *are* us. We are them. So we try to control our thoughts, repress our feelings and change our behaviour to match our mood. We project a certain identity according to what we think other people want from us. Since our changes are based on a faulty reading of others and ourselves, this is almost certain to lead to problems.

This *sūtra* teaches us that thoughts, feelings, mind, emotion, memory, imagination, our beliefs about who we are and our roles in life are all essential parts of ourselves, but they are also the workings of ego. We have either inherited them, created them or learned them from others. They are part of the changeable world of matter. They come and go. We can intervene to make them stronger or dial them down, and realizing that we have this control is so empowering.

Our essence is something else, something higher and deeper. This deep consciousness is unchanging and is part of the non-material, subtle world. I think of it as the essence of 'you-ness', that hard-to-define quality that makes you a unique individual.

When we assume that the activities of our egos add up to our real selves, this fundamental misunderstanding leads to other problems: our desires, aversions and fears.

So how can we reduce the working of ego yet keep our personality? By calling it what it is. By understanding that, though it has our best interests at heart, it also has a tendency to be a little domineering. If we're living through a significant change, such as becoming a parent, for example, this shift in identity might feel really destabilizing. When this happens, our egos surge up, insisting they can help us out by defining a new role and replacing our identity as quickly as possible. 'Who am I if I'm not a party girl?' your ego might be screaming inside. 'I'm a mother now? OK . . . I've got this. I'm a mother . . .' Ego loves to supply a new crutch to replace the old one. It loves to fix our problems for us, even if it might actually be useful and healthy to sit with the problem a while. Take a look at it from various angles . . . Consider whether it's not really a problem at all but an opportunity.

When was the last time you felt your ego surge up? What triggered it? What did it feel like and what were the consequences? Did you blame yourself or others? Did you create excuses? Can you begin to identify the rules that you'd put in place, and how when they were broken, that triggered the upset? Can you see how you might adapt those rules to make an ego flare-up less likely?

Ultimately, when you embrace not-knowing as the only real and realistic state of mind, you align with your essence to stand up to your ego. This isn't easy. It takes practice. But there's so much more to you than your monkey mind or your messy feelings. You just have to trust that it's there and practise moving towards it.

First, though, we need to know more about the other *kleśa* . . .

Hardwired to want more – of everything (2.7)

It's perhaps the oldest human flaw: the desire for more, whether it's more knowledge, more money or more power. We want more of everything that we find pleasing and we also want better: a better job, better clothes, a better body, a better partner or life. Every religion and philosophy talks about the thirst for more and tries to show people how dangerous and damaging it is. Humanity remains stubbornly incapable of knowing when enough is enough.

Modern biology has revealed the workings of the reward circuit in our brain and shown that we are hardwired to desire things that make us feel good, even if the reward is temporary and the effect is harmful in the long term. But you don't need to be a neuroscientist to know that too much of a good but addictive thing leaves you dependent and weakened. You just need to have found yourself scrolling Instagram late at night instead of going to bed. Again. Or promising yourself you'll only drink at weekends and then having a glass of wine on a Thursday because it's practically the weekend and next week on Wednesday and the week after on Tuesday because why not, everyone needs a little treat at the end of the day.

Alternatively, you could read the *Yoga Sūtra*, which identified excessive attachment to things that only briefly make us happy as a big problem more than 3,000 years ago. Thinking that getting what we want over and over again will continue to bring us the same happiness it did the first time, is deluded. Satisfying our desires can only ever feel good for a moment. Trying to make that moment permanent leads to problems.

I once worked with a gentleman who had made a very advantageous marriage when he was young. His bride was a wealthy woman, they had a family, she adored him. It was never enough for him. He left that marriage and, though he's remained wealthy, he has never settled with a new partner. Yet he keeps on looking for love. Sadly, he admitted to me that it had become clear to him that he had been happier during his marriage than at any other point in his life.

He's not unusual. It's all very well to point out that being led by desire can get us into trouble. Most of us know that, at least in theory. The problem lies in calibrating how much desire is appropriate. How much of anything is enough? Is this as good as it gets or is there something better out there, and, if so, why settle?

These are difficult questions with no definite answers. We can only hope to tackle them with confidence if we develop the clarity, comfort and stability we need to assess our reality as it is. And if we are humble enough (clear-sighted enough) to acknowledge that none of us is immune to the pull of desire.

It's important to learn the difference between motivation, ambition and desire. After all, if we never wanted to achieve something, or to set ourselves a goal, our lives would be the poorer. The way I understand these calibrations is that motivation is the state of being ready and willing to take on a challenge. It's essential and positive. When ego links up with motivation we get ambition, which is beginning to pull us into potentially dangerous territory. Our ego, as we've seen, loves to convince us it's doing us a favour while actually draining away our essence. And desire is motivation on steroids. Unstoppable, always hungry for more. The only way to dial our desires down is to interrupt them. Question them. Sit with them a little.

The more we do this, the more clearly we see what it is we really want. Sometimes, for example, we think we are yearning for a new romantic partner when actually that yearning could be satisfied by going deeper into the situation or relationship that we're in already. It's fine to want change, but perhaps change the relationship, not the person? Sometimes, we confuse what we want with what we need. It's often easier to start afresh with a new partner than learn the art of diving deeper with somebody. Until six months down the line we find ourselves in the same spot.

Ask yourself, 'What is it that I really want?' And is that desire blinding you to something you need? Do you have the courage to fight against weaknesses?

After desire and before fear comes loathing (2.8)

Is there something you really can't tolerate? I'm not thinking so much of a dislike of spiders, more an inability to sit still without scrolling or a tendency to take well-meant comments as vicious personal criticism. Perhaps it's a person you can't stand. Your colleague? A member of your family?

Anything that triggers a strong aversion has a lot of power over us. Just like excessive attachment, unreasonable aversion enfeebles us, makes us less than we might be. Our aversions are usually fuelled by painful memories. You might overreact to criticism from your boss, for example, because it reminds you of being endlessly criticized by a parent or a teacher. As always, misunderstanding is at the root of the problem here. Your boss is not your teacher. You are not living the same moment. You are a different person now and could react to the criticism differently if you could only reduce the discomfort your aversion provokes.

The outcomes of aversion are not pretty. We get angry, or we become consumed with jealousy. We might even feel hatred. These states are uncomfortable and destabilizing. They might cause us to behave in ways that we don't recognize. Perhaps we lash out, verbally or physically. Or we withdraw contact or affection. Naturally this is likely to trigger an equally negative reaction. The net result is conflict, and worse – we have given away our comfort and stability by allowing aversion to drop us into hate or jealousy.

But, as with everything, there's an opportunity here. Aversion is triggered by a constriction in your heart. That tightness is desperate for relief. It's calling to you, trying to get your attention so that you recognize it, see it from a different angle, release it. Aversion is an opportunity to heal.

What (or whom) do you strongly dislike? What (or whom) are you jealous of? What are you holding on to so tightly that's behind the feeling? How is it keeping you trapped or how is it fuelling you? Don't push these uncomfortable feelings away. Take a closer look at them. Can you imagine doing something different with these feelings and that energy?

Fear is the biggie, even for the wisest person (2.9)

Our final *kleśa* is fear, and anxiety arises from fear. And here we're up against a big challenge, because to be human is to live with the knowledge that we all have something to lose. We may be destitute and without a friend in the world, but as long as we're alive, we're still in the game.

Most of us are, of course, blessedly fortunate. We each have a roof over our head and food on the table. We have family or friends or both; health, hope, purpose or possibility. To imagine losing these things can be profoundly anxiety-inducing and I am not going to pretend otherwise.

But yoga is encouraging us to face our fears with more calm and firmness. It shows us that, when we feel anxious, rather than getting swirled away into a chain of panicky thoughts, a better response could be to ask what we're frightened of losing. And is that threat real, right here and now? Slowing down and asking these questions can help with even the big existential fears. You may be frightened of dying, but if – right now – you're fit and well and looking after yourself, and taking sensible decisions about your health and your behaviour, then your fear is based on a projection into the future. Yes, you will die, but you are not dying yet. Don't let fear obscure the reality of the life you have right now.

Fear is challenging. We are all at the mercy of our fight-or-flight response, the hardwired reaction to perceived threat that evolved to keep us safe from predators but now makes us panic at every e-mail from our boss. But we can strengthen our resilience to fears and insecurities. Especially the not-so-existential ones. The fear of failure and what other people think of us, the fretting about saying something stupid or whether we're too old to wear shorts and whether we're a good enough mother/

father/colleague/yogi . . . All those everyday insecurities may feel very real, but they are just the work of our imagination, stuck in a groove of speculation and catastrophizing. 'What if she hates me, what if I don't pass, what if I lose my job, what if I screw it up, what if this and that and . . . ?' These 'what if's have no part in our lives. And the practice of yoga shows us how to lessen their joy-sucking hold on us. (If you're struggling with anxiety there's an exercise on page 155 that will support you with this.)

There's a webinar I love to watch by Stanford University biologist Robert Sapolsky that never fails to make me smile, given my close brush with mortality: 'Why Zebras Don't Get Ulcers: Stress & Health'. The *Yoga Sūtra* can teach us how to be more like the zebra. Meanwhile, let's go back to looking at the *kleśa* in the round.

> *Ask yourself, 'What is it I'm scared of losing, right now? Is my fear based on my current reality or is it a work of imagination? A projection into the future? What's really going on here?'*

Dealing with kleśa*: before or after, but not during* (2.10)

Imagine you're cycling home, minding your own business, when some guy cuts you up. Idiot! He drives off, then drops back and at the roundabout he cuts you up *again*. For a second you can't quite believe it. You're frozen in disbelief. This guy is the biggest idiot in town.

What do you do? At this moment, all outcomes are still possible because you haven't yet reacted. You could observe the guy being an idiot, mentally step back, realize it has nothing to do with you and literally move on. But maybe you're freaked by the close shave. Your heart is pounding. You're angry. Insulted. Who does this guy think he is? You can still see him, so you race up behind and give him the finger. He leans out the window and hurls a torrent of abuse. You arrive home in a foul mood, vent to your partner, fail to ask them how their day's been, respond angrily when they accuse you of dumping a load of toxic mood on them the second you walk through the door, have a full-blown row and only half an hour later recall that moment when you could still have nipped everything in the bud, back at the roundabout, by saying to yourself, 'That was unpleasant, but I'm OK and none of this guy's behaviour has anything to do with me.'

It is one of the few iron laws of yoga that none of us can deal with the negative consequences of *kleśa* once we've stumbled into them and been swept up in their emotional turmoil. You have an opportunity, right up until the fear or anger or desire breaks, to detach from it, observe it and step away. But once you're in the middle of its chaos, there is nothing you can do but go with it until it passes. Only afterwards, when it's died down, can you take a look at whatever action and reactions occurred and calmly try to find a different perspective. Maybe the guy is still a jerk, but that doesn't mean you are. And actually, perhaps your partner had a point.

The art of nipping the manifestations of *kleśa* in the bud is what we're all in training for, throughout our lives. It is really hard to do when we're starting out on our yoga journey and impossible to pull off every time, even with decades of practice. It's such an amazing life skill, though, and can save so much aggression, heartbreak, misunderstanding and missed opportunity. It's really worth practising. And in the meantime, as the next *sūtra* tells us, the hindsight route is always available to us mere mortals. It is one of our key tools for learning in yoga. Practise getting comfortable with looking back over spiralling situations and searching for the moment when you felt the emotional reaction generated by *kleśa* surge in you. Reflect, meditate and imagine how it could have gone differently.

When did you last have an opportunity to nip a spiralling emotional reaction in the bud? Did you manage to take it, or did you watch yourself in the situation and miss it? Could you have done anything differently? How did you reflect on it afterwards? Why didn't you act when you could have done? Please don't blame yourself or anybody else at any point during this questioning.

Get comfortable with not knowing (2.11)

Now that you know a little more about how *kleśa* can generate problems, it's time to return to their primary source. Remember that, actually, not having a clue what's going on – either in *your* head or in other people's – is the basic condition of human life. We all struggle to understand and to do the right thing. We all make mistakes based on our faulty perception. We do it every single day and, honestly, that's fine. Being aware that when *kleśa* are driving things we'll find it difficult to wrest back control of the steering is a huge and powerful start. It also takes practice to build the ability, agility and awareness to nip it in the bud, and that's fine too.

Once you've begun to get comfortable with these notions, you're also ready to start doing something about things after the event. Ever so gently, with patience and curiosity, you can begin to dial down the power and heat and noise of the problems that sprout from the roots of *kleśa*.

How? That's what we're moving on to now, via a jump to a different section of the *Yoga Sūtra*. But the short answer is: meditation. Which is to say, yoga is the key to successfully battling *kleśa*.

Without attributing instant blame to yourself or others, and without listing excuses to justify behaviours, go back over a situation that's caused you a problem. Step back from your involvement and your notion of right and wrong on your part or theirs. Where in this interaction could you have done something differently? What were the feelings that gave you the signal? Have you been here before? Can you trust your feeling so you can take responsibility and do something differently in future?

Group 3: Prepare to practise

There are three important principles to bear in mind when we begin to practise yoga. The first is that success is entirely possible, but it does take effort. The effort is rewarding in itself, but it's also demanding, and there are no shortcuts. When I say 'success', I am thinking in life – not in yoga. We have success when our yoga practice supports us to experience fewer of the difficulties that arise from unchecked *kleśa*, and to live more comfortably and with greater awareness and purpose.

The second principle is that linear progression is not a useful way to think about developing. It's essential to let go of the notion that, for example, doing an hour a day of yoga practice entitles us to feel serene all the time or to 'get better' at yoga. There's no such thing as being 'bad' or 'good' at yoga, because success is measured not by your body's flexibility in *āsana* but by an increased capacity to live your life comfortably. Remember also that slog is as bad for the heart, mind and body as laziness. The right amount of effort, neither more nor less, is what's required. How can you tell how much is the right amount for you? Through practice.

The third important principle is that practising yoga doesn't mean you will escape the endless flow of life's challenges. None of us can prevent stuff from coming at us. All we can do is practise honing our responses, knowing that we will still make mistakes along the way. That's not a failure, it's just the way the world works, and we work within it. Our relationship with ourselves and with other people is the ground where we practise being comfortable and stable despite the chaos.

Take responsibility for all your actions, beginning with your practice (2.1)

One of the most fundamental lessons in life is that only a few things are under our control. Most are not. Being able to distinguish which is which is the difference between misery and happiness.

Broadly speaking, other people – and what they say, do or choose – are not under your control. Your actions and reactions *are* within your control, and you need to take responsibility for them. Nobody else can do this for you, and if you don't do it, you will never fulfil your potential for happiness, success, personal growth, spiritual development or anything else that makes life interesting and worthwhile. But if this sounds like a heavy-duty struggle, remember that the responsibility is also an endless opportunity to bring about positive change. Every single action or reaction that you experience offers a chance to change something in your life for the better.

This *sūtra* has three important components. The requirement to act, to do something. The importance of reflection, to observe with reduced judgement. And the ability to be ready to accept, understand what it is we need to move on and not fall in a trap again. It's asking you to practise the habit of taking responsibility for your actions. As we've just seen, learning to reflect honestly on yourself is fundamental to yoga. This process also helps you to see other people's actions from different perspectives and begin to accept. This is yoga in action.

But thinking back over things, though crucial, is only one part of yoga practice. We can't theorize about how to change our feelings or relate to someone. We will achieve change only through action, through *doing*. That's how we learn. So, reflection does not imply rumination, passively accepting what's happened or turning it over and inflating it in our minds afterwards. Reflection, combined with genuine acceptance, is part of an active yoga practice and is a path to greater self-awareness. And, given that all we can control in this life are our own thoughts and feelings, self-awareness is pretty important.

Where are your strengths and weaknesses in doing things, thinking and accepting? Is one greater than the others? Are you missing one? Ask yourself whether you have a tendency to overthink things or rush in without enough thinking. Do you accept things the way they are? Or can't you accept and constantly question or resist them? None of these approaches is wrong as such, but any and all of them might lead to problems. How can all three of these form part of one healthy interaction for you? Understanding the particular ways we get ourselves into trouble is crucial to steering away from it in future.

Less hurt, more ease and more you-ness . . . eventually (2.2)

This is an important line in my reading of the *Yoga Sūtra*. It's a promise that we're on our way to a life of less struggle and conflict, and more contentment. We're working with the cycle of yoga in action. We're heading for a taste of who we truly are. There's a certain amount of faith involved because we're never going to escape the chaos of life, no matter how much yoga we practise, and we won't always be sure that we're moving in the right direction. So this *sūtra* advises us to take our time. Get to know what works and what doesn't. As our understanding deepens, it will be easier to integrate what we learn on our yoga mat or during *prāṇāyāma* (pronounced pra-nai-yah-ma), or breathwork, into our lives.

For example, you might begin to see that you don't need to strain your body or breath in order to feel a benefit. In fact, pushing too hard causes a sense of discomfort. Perhaps you don't need to strain or push to feel happy in your relationship, either. Or maybe you discover that unless you practise every day you don't learn anything. Perhaps it's time to step up your efforts at college or work as well. I'm not saying that there's necessarily any direct correlation between effort in one area of life and another. It's more that using yoga to interrogate *how* we do things, and what results we get, might open our eyes to other dimensions in which we could ask the same questions and uncover useful insights.

One thing is certain: the more you practise yoga in action, the easier it is to reduce the impact of the five *kleśa* (not-knowing, ego, desire, aversion, fear). Your ego quietens down. You cling less because you're less afraid. You indulge yourself less because you're less wrapped up in your needs. So we could think of this line as a reminder that, while it's a misunderstanding to imagine we'll ever outwit our difficulties entirely, we *can* hope for improvement over time. If we don't feel any easing of our tight back or sad heart, however gradual, we might want to try a different yoga tool.

For me, what this *sūtra* shows us is that the promise of yoga is not reaching some mystical higher plane. It's more about experiencing less distress and feeling stable and comfortable enough to simply enjoy being ourselves. Yoga returns us to ourselves. Once we've grasped this, we're truly ready to begin.

Ask yourself, 'What's easing for me? Am I becoming more aware of which things hurt me? Could I say that I am feeling "more myself"?'

Group 4: The foundation: how our mind can be hurtful or not hurtful

The opening four lines of the *Yoga Sūtra* are a beautiful invitation to understand yoga as a state of mind unlike any other. It is not one that we can move directly into. Yoga is almost a by-product of three aspects of consciousness operating simultaneously: being present in the here and now, paying full attention and being motivated to change. When we combine these states of mind, yoga is the result.

The text describes yoga by contrasting it with different states of mind, different kinds of mind as well as the participation of mental activities. These everyday mental activities, such as day-dreaming, analysing, fretting and ruminating, are the ones that take up most of our time and energy. They are natural, unavoidable parts of human life and can be beneficial, but they can also hold us back and keep us low. The more time and energy we spend on developing a yoga state of mind and the less time we spend on superfluous mental activity, the more space we create for change.

Are you ready and motivated? (1.1)

In this fabulous line, which invites and welcomes us into the ongoing conversation, the *Yoga Sūtra* asks us if we're ready and motivated to participate. Do we want to grow? Are we really, truly here, in this moment, ready and willing to start? Because, actually, that readiness and that motivation are prerequisites – our conditions of entry into the process of investigation we're embarking on. Some of us are ready, though not motivated. Others are motivated but not ready. We need to be both, in order to have awareness, be present and evolve.

The sense I get in this line is that, as well as the invitation, there is a clarification: your life *can* change, but you have to be ready and up for whatever is about to happen.

Do you feel ready? Do you feel up for the challenge? Right here in this moment, can you imagine feeling calm and alert at the same time? Where are you, right now? What are you feeling? Are you able to create even a tiny space between the essential you and the busy-mind you? That could be as simple as noting that now you're not sure you know what I'm on about, when a minute ago you were feeling comfortable and positive!

Enveloping vs *grasping and unfocused* (1.2)

Yoga is a by-product of our ability to maintain a particular kind of link with (or keep our attention on) an object. The fundamental link in question is between the perceiver (you), and what's being perceived (an object). This is done through what does the perceiving (the mind and senses). In order to cultivate a yoga mindset, we need first to recognize that there is a difference between that part of ourselves which is able to perceive our thoughts or feelings, and the thoughts and feelings being perceived. Even mental events, from abstract thought to gut feeling, are part of the material world – objects to be perceived. They are qualitatively different from the essential part of us – the subtle 'you' – that is doing the perceiving.

Having recognized the difference between who we really are and the thoughts and feelings that run around our minds, we next need to cultivate a certain kind of link between them. That link is a quality of attention that is expansive rather than brittle and enveloping rather than grasping.

We often think that paying attention means focusing intently on a single object, but attention in yoga is not about laser-like grasp. It's softer, broader and multidimensional. It's like a rewarding and relaxed conversation between two friends in a café, one that's so absorbing that both people can look up and say, 'Yes, please, I'd love another coffee,' to the server and then slip straight back into the stream of their chat. Yoga is what happens when we're able to sit in the middle of life's chaos and pay calm, relaxed, enveloping attention to everything that comes up.

To understand this is to know something of the difference between activities of the mind (such as worrying about a job interview or solving an equation) and your deeper consciousness, the essence of you-ness. The *Yoga Sūtra* calls this deeper, clearer enveloping mind *citta*, and contrasts it with the other kinds or qualities of mind. When we are practising yoga, the mind is not engaged in intellectual activity or indulging in sensory experience. It's not asleep or stuck in rumination or obsessing about its own needs and wants. It's not egocentric. It's capable of taking what it observes or learns and integrating that, enveloping that, within itself.

As well as these different *kinds* of mind, the *Yoga Sūtra* shows us that there is a spectrum of energetic *states* of mind, ranging from heavy and lethargic at one end to manic and jumpy at the other. We are invited to begin to recognize all these different flavours of activity. Many of us are blind to the mental, emotional and energetic activity that's constantly shifting inside us. We might be unaware that we've become agitated until we fly off the handle, for example. We might not notice we're overthinking a problem until our friend asks us a question for the third time. The more we recognize these flavours of our internal workings, the easier it is to enjoy and cultivate the yoga mind.

Tomorrow, see if you can identify some of your states and kinds of mind. (A state could be agitated, heavy, normal, distracted, focused. A kind could be sensory, intellectual – stuck in your head, egotistical.) You don't need to use specific labels unless you want to. Just try to get a feel for when you're problem-solving, say, or when you're soothing your mind with distractions. When are you feeding your senses, your sight, smell, taste etc.? When are you trying to gratify your ego in some way? Remember, none of these things is bad and you don't need to judge yourself. This is the wonder of the mind.

More of what makes you 'you' (1.3)

This super calm and positive *sūtra* offers us a promise. It's telling us, in a simple and reassuring way, that if we achieve more of our yoga quality of mind – this enveloping, encompassing, expansive mind – and spend less time on the other kinds, then the essence of our being will have more opportunity to shine.

You know those mornings when you're tired and grumpy and desperate for the first cup of coffee? You walk past a coffee shop and it smells amazing, but you're already a bit late to work so you don't go in, and now all you can think about is how much you want a coffee, how much you need one, deserve one, and what will happen if you can't get one . . . You're obsessed with the coffee, which is not so bad since it's only a coffee and, hey, you'll probably snap out of this spiral of coffee thoughts soon enough, one way or another, but it's still almost as if your mind has been taken over for a while.

Sometimes, however, this spiralling thinking and obsessive feeling and wanting is more serious. Not just in terms of the hook that hauls us in, which can be a genuinely addictive substance or pastime, but because whatever it is we're fussing over simply isn't worth it. Many of us lose long chunks of time and waste vast amounts of mental and emotional energy on obsessive thoughts that distract us from more important and interesting ones. We can literally lose connection with who we are.

It doesn't have to be that way. More you-ness is available to you and yoga is a way towards it.

> *When you are happily in the flow of living your life, what does this success look like? What is the result?*

Most of what we consider as reality isn't real (1.4)

This might sound a little out there, but I don't mean that the world you can touch and smell doesn't exist, or that there's no such thing as agreed-upon reality, or that facts and truth don't matter. It's more that most of our personal worldview – how we think about things and what we believe – is the result of our interpretations and projections. For example, a red car is just a red car, but whether red-car drivers are fun-loving extroverts or tacky show-offs is a matter of opinion. Our opinions are the end result of long processes of analysis and assessment by our sensory mind, our intellectual mind, our ego-driven mind, our identity – all those different kinds of mind we saw just now. They all have their particular angle on everything we encounter. When you put them all together you get the set of opinions and expectations, biases and projections that each one of us calls reality.

Now, there's nothing wrong with this as such. Human beings construct their own worldviews out of all the material they find lying around: from what they've inherited, from their lived experience, what their parents showed them, what they were taught in school and learned from their mates and so on. The first point to make is that these projections we call reality will either help or hinder us. If, for example, you have constructed a view that insists that yoga is just for girls or Christmas must always be spent with your parents, then an upset to these projections of your ego-driven mind and identity-based mind might end up getting you into trouble. Such views are not necessarily wrong, but they're not necessarily the truth, either; they're just *your* truth. And they are constructed by the rules that you've put in place in your mind.

And the even bigger point is that if we can't recognize the

difference between *another's* truth and *our* truth, we're going to struggle with all the nuance of this wonderful world we live in. We're going to end up telling ourselves stories that don't serve us and create expectations that will set us up for a fall.

The enveloped and enveloping mind of someone in a state of yoga, on the other hand, is less prone to jumping to the wrong conclusion or imagining the worst. It is better at learning from experience and releasing attachments. It can hold something very lightly, cradle it and absorb it. It is a state of absolute comfort and stability no matter what it's presented with.

Can you identify some of your projections that have morphed into beliefs or rules? I'm not thinking of society's moral and ethical rules about decent behaviour, more a personal rule like that one about Christmas. It could be a silly thing or a big one. Search for something you assume is 'normal' or 'just the way things happen', either about the world or about yourself.

Everyday minds are either useful or not (1.5)

What, specifically, are our minds up to when they're serving the needs of our egos or our identities or our senses or our intellect rather than the essence of who we really are? What might they be doing, either sluggishly or skittishly, depending on the energy of our minds?

This is one of the most empowering lines in the *Yoga Sūtra*. Very simply it's saying that all your mental activities are either hurtful or not. It's something to reflect on again and again, and in every situation you find yourself in daily life. It's referring to your perception and how you construct it. How you perceive things in this world, including yourself. And this is the very art (and heart) of yoga. Is it that you now have or always have had a choice? Or is it by you now knowing this you have an opportunity?

Take Jay, who is mid-thirties, wants to meet someone to settle down with and is on all the dating apps. Jay spends at least an hour each day replying to and vetting matches, messaging and organizing dates. It's easy to get lots of dates and regular hook-ups, though they never lead to success in a relationship. What is going wrong? Jay is good-looking, gets on with everyone, is in great shape – works out regularly, owns a home, travels often . . . you get the picture. But it's just not happening. Jay tells me that, either immediately, or after a week, or maybe after a month at most, every potential partner gets dropped because of some fault that has surfaced. They're toast. So we start investigating. We need to understand how the *kleśa* are behind the way the minds of people like Jay work; how the excuses they use to protect against getting hurt are actually hurtful to them. How they use blame to do the same, and what are the techniques and patterns they're using to distract from entering into a deeper healthy relationship.

So here we have it – another really important component of yoga. We understand that the mental activities we have are part of us and always will be. They're either hurtful or not. Depending on our state of mind and kind of mind, they're involved somewhere in our perception with more or less influence. As we'll discover, there's no getting away from them, they exist even in a yoga state of mind.

> *Can it be possible that something that hurts us now won't hurt us again? What justifications and excuses do we put in place to protect our perception of something? Can you begin to imagine a different set of rules to live by?*

Admiring the playing field of projection (1.6)

In this line, the *Yoga Sūtra* defines the mind by listing its everyday activities. There are five of them and, as we have seen, they can all be helpful or harmful, leading either to beneficial effects or to problems. The five activities are: correct comprehension, misunderstanding, imagination, sleep and memory. These are the basic building blocks of all mental activity. They keep our minds busy ticking over or plunge us into rest, depending on the need of the moment, but none of them brings us closer to yoga. They can produce a sort of internal chaos. Yoga begins to occur when we get some clarity on how we identify with that chaos.

Most of us find it difficult to detach from the workings of memory and imagination. We tend to get lost in nostalgia or in fantasy. As for correct comprehension, we may grasp something fleetingly, but then it slips away again into misunderstanding. And even sleep, that fetish of the wellness industry, can get us into trouble if we sleep too little or too much, or just obsess about the amount we're getting.

We invent stories or rules as a way of managing the pitfalls created by these activities of our minds. Then we fall for the 'truth' of our projections. Changing them would be painful and difficult, so we mostly don't. We prefer to remain stable even if it's uncomfortable. But all progress, evolution, creativity and healing is dependent on questioning these constructs. I firmly believe that the ability to recognize and seize an opportunity to try a new angle on an old story is the cornerstone of success in our lives.

Can we just pause here and admire the view? Aren't our minds incredible? They construct a world of our very own for us to exist in. That's kind of impressive, even if it means that sometimes we're wandering in a hall of mirrors. The *Yoga Sūtra* is clear that there is nothing wrong with how we think and feel in our everyday lives. It's not that rumination or daydreaming or wanting another piece of chocolate cake is inherently bad and must be eradicated. (Which is handy, because most of us are never going to manage it, and life would be pretty dull if we did.)

In order to feel more comfortable and stable we do not need to eradicate anything – we simply need to bring more awareness to our desires, fears and aversions, as well as the difference between *another's* truth and *our* truth. In this way we can create enough distance so that the chocolate cake (or the fear of failure, or the shouty inner critic) doesn't win out every time. We can start to see past the stage-set our minds have built and notice a bit more of everything else that's going on around us. That's good enough.

So let's stop and admire the view we've created. Rather than criticize our minds for simply doing their jobs, let's appreciate them. It's not a question of yoga 'the good guy', versus all these baddies. Every aspect of mind is on the same team.

Celebrate your mind's successes. Can you think of a moment when you suddenly understood something or someone? When you were able to change a habit that had been annoying you or leave a relationship that no longer served you? What about the last time you learned a new skill? Our minds are amazing and work constantly on our behalf.

Don't mistake your cleverness for true understanding (1.7)

'Correct comprehension' sounds great, but it is different from the understanding that occurs in a state of yoga. Comprehension, as a gross mental activity, is an output of your brain's processing and analysis of the information it constantly receives. From a direct experience incoming signals are captured by your eyes, ears, mouth, nose and skin and passed along to your brain, which uses memory and imagination to interpret the information – it infers. The brain then cracks on with solving problems, drawing comparisons, inventing and creating – referencing to what it knows and believes. Brilliant – except it's prone to error, as we've already seen. Bias, positive and negative associations, over-attachment to being right:

your intellectual brain is amazing but limited. Only when we practise the enveloping attention and self-reflection of yoga do we get closer to seeing things (people, ourselves) as they really are, and acting accordingly.

But that's only the first step towards true understanding. In order to evaluate something correctly we need to bear in mind that the context may have changed since the last time we looked at anything similar. During a Covid lockdown I was talking to a client about his financial worries. He was running a business providing short academic courses online. He was struggling. He told me that he wasn't converting interest to sales in anything like the usual way. He'd recently advertised a taster session on Facebook that 350 signed up to. On the day, 100 people attended online. But only three of them signed up for the course. 'What am I doing wrong?' he wanted to know. 'Is it Covid? People feeling the pinch financially? Or is it me? This time last year I was a success; now, I'm a failure.' He was stuck in a cycle of worry, rumination and ego-bound obsession over success, and he couldn't correctly comprehend that this was both an opportunity and a requirement to do something different.

I suggested he detach from believing that this was a problem he could crack alone, through his powers of analysis. I invited him to see that he'd had huge success at the first two stages of his process: 350 people interested; 100 people on the day. Could he repeat those two stages with an open mind about what stage three would look like? Everything has changed. Hold another event and ask his attendees what they want. If he could get comfortable with not knowing what the *new* correct evaluation of his situation was, I was sure it would emerge.

We tend to get attached to our identity as a smart person, as somebody who can spot opportunities or do a deal or work things out. If we have a certain amount of success we tell ourselves a story about where that success came from, which lays down a template for how we handle the next similar situation. Often, the story stars us as the hero of correct comprehension. If our story falters, that can feel very destabilizing.

Yoga insists that, to be really successful, we need to demonstrate our ability to comprehend correctly not once or twice but over and over again, across many different circumstances. In order to do this, we need to be able to draw on three different sources to boost our understanding: firstly, the direct personal experience that is prioritized in yoga; secondly, the power of inference; and thirdly, everything we learn from external authorities that we trust, which might range from a governing body or legal structure, to our parents' teachings or to those of religion. Relying on any one of these sources alone will eventually get us into trouble. Using a combination, and in the right mix for each situation, will bring far more success.

It's this adaptability that kicks correct comprehension up a notch – it's either hurtful or not – nothing more. Great things happen when we combine our analysis of what we've experienced with reflection, detach from our need to be the hero and invite help from others. If we can do all that, we open up to receiving an education in life.

Can you break down how you correctly understand something into three components: direct experience, inference and reference sources. What mix do you have? Why? How much do you rely on one and not so much the others? How can you increase the influence of one or more? How could you use all three together?

Your mistakes are just more opportunities (1.8)

Most of us are absolutely wedded to our core belief that 95 per cent of the time we're in the right and it's the other person who's in the wrong. And yet, in this line, the *Yoga Sūtra* gently points out that misunderstanding is the most common of the mental activities.

I find this immensely reassuring. We're all just struggling to figure things out, getting it wrong and dealing (badly) with the consequences. This is entirely normal and there's no point in beating ourselves up about it. That won't make us feel more comfortable or more stable. A more productive response is to try to get better at recognizing our misunderstandings in time to do something about them. There is an internal feeling that comes with misunderstanding.

The other morning at the stables, Sarah, the assistant, was telling me about my horse's mood, as she always does. She made a suggestion about how to handle her. 'Try *x*, because when she's in this mood she does *y*,' Sarah said to me.

I responded by saying, 'I know.'

I could tell the moment I saw Sarah's face that she'd taken my response as arrogant dismissal rather than acknowledgement of her infinitely greater experience of riding in general and this horse in particular. And fair enough. As soon as I said it, I saw I'd phrased my answer clumsily, and accidentally given offence. I hadn't been paying enough attention to our conversation. I was concentrating on the horse. Sarah and I don't yet know each other well, so misunderstandings are more likely.

Fortunately, I noticed what I'd done. Not in time to nip my remark in the bud but still close enough to make an apology easy to give and easier to accept. I also said what I should have said the first time, which was, 'Thanks, that's a good idea.' Sarah was gracious enough to say sorry to me for having made a mistake herself, when she misinterpreted my intent. I went off for my ride and tried to put into practice what Sarah had advised. No harm done.

Sometimes, of course, the stakes are far higher and the consequences of our actions much harder to resolve, which perhaps helps to explain why many of us are so frightened of making mistakes. It can help to remind ourselves that everyone makes them – literally, everyone – and they make a lot of them. They're either hurtful to us or not. We are not failing when we take something the wrong way or cock up at work; we are simply being human. Rather than indulging in melodramatic stories of self-reproach or guilt, we can take responsibility, offer an apology and reflect on our misunderstanding in order to try to do better next time. As the *Yoga Sūtra* would have it, that's enough.

The next time you realize that there's been a misunderstanding, can you seize the opportunity it presents? Rather than cover it up and carry on, could you pause, point it out or admit it – without recrimination – and see what happens next. In this way you will gain an opportunity to learn something, either about the other person or about yourself.

Imagination: yoga turns it into a superpower (1.9)

Our ability to imagine the future, to dream and create, is both a gift and a curse. It's a gift to be able to create something out of nothing, and we all do it every day. We plan a conversation ahead of time. We imagine what it will feel like to meet up with our partner at the weekend. We create stories, paint pictures on canvas or in our minds.

But imagination can also steal our creative power. It can steal our ability to imagine our way towards a clearer understanding. It can be damaging, hollow and deceiving. If our imagination tends to conjure up fearful visions of what might happen in the future, we end up anxious. If it leads us to dwell in a fantasy detached from reality, we end up living a lie, coveting what we don't have or feeling inadequate. We imagine what if.

Imagination is the driver of all change; if we cannot imagine the difference we wish to create, we will never achieve it. And if we don't do something with the creative force that surges within every one of us, there is a danger it will become malevolent. I believe that anxiety is very often thwarted creativity, and if you are being creative you can't be anxious at the same time.

I don't hold much with the platitudes of positive thinking, but I do believe that imagination needs positivity to keep it on course. Yoga helps us to understand, appreciate and direct our imagination for good. It supports us to mix our imagination with just a dash of ego and desire to produce creativity, rather than mix it with fear, which results in anxiety or hostility.

Our imagination will always extend what we know and lead us on into our future. When we practise yoga we send our imagination in the right direction for us.

> *Can you think of a time when your ability to imagine a positive outcome helped you realize it? What about a time when your imagination hurt or hindered you? Can you can recall any conversations during which a particular word or point pulled you out of the present moment and either back into the past or forward into the future? In either case, it's your imagination that led you. Was that a good direction for you, or not?*

Sleep is golden, but a heavy mind will get you down (1.10)

Does anybody else think that, lately, we've become obsessed with sleep? It is, of course, fundamental to good health, but some of us fret so much over whether we're getting enough that we ruin our chances of nodding off. It might seem that a troubled relationship with sleep is a very modern concern, but the *Yoga Sūtra* identified it as a surprisingly slippery subject way back when.

According to yoga, sleep is the opposite of the meditative state. In sleep, the you that does the perceiving withdraws from activity of any kind. It curls in on itself in order to be alone, to allow the mind, body and senses to rest and recuperate. This is crucial for both mind and body, but sleep's inertia is a risk if it seeps into our waking minds. As a parallel, if mental busyness intrudes into sleep, that is also a problem.

The transitions between sleep and wakefulness can be tricky for many of us. Transitions always are. We're probably all familiar with the phenomenon of feeling exhausted but being unable to nod off because our brain is racing. Our mind chugs through what we did that day or the to-do list for tomorrow, and we can't switch off. In the morning we might struggle to get up and get going.

These sensations are certainly uncomfortable, and a consistent lack of sleep is definitely bad for our mental and physical health. Ask any parent of a young child how stable and comfortable they feel, and they'll probably hurl some choice words in your direction.

But actually, for the rest of us, sleep problems such as insomnia or violent nightmares are – you guessed it – a learning opportunity. When we sleep, we slip away from rule-bound reality into a domain where our minds do whatever they need in order to process what they've taken in. Yoga tells us that, although sleep needn't obsess us, it is worth being curious about. And it's definitely worth smoothing our transitions into and out of it. This is why I find it crucial to practise yoga when I wake and when I am preparing for bed. In fact, it's as close as I get to a universal rule: practise ten minutes as soon as possible after waking and ten minutes last thing at night. In the morning this helps to prepare for the day. In the evening it helps to prepare for sleep.

What can you learn about how you wind down at the end of the day? The rules you apply to the sleep you think you should have? How you deal with sleep if you are tired or agitated? The next time you experience waking in the night, can you speak kindly to your mind rather than angrily? Look not to get over-involved with your fear that you won't get enough sleep, and instead reassure your mind that you're grateful, it's doing a good job and carry on.

Beautiful minds dancing through time (I.11)

The final mental activity is memory, which is fundamental to our sense of who we are. Without memory there could be no sorting, analysis and archiving of the information our brain receives from the world. So both perception and the construction of our reality depend on memory. And memory is at work in laying down the patterns of behaviour that we see in ourselves and in others, patterns that eventually solidify into our projected personality and sense of identity.

But in yoga, memory is not just a cognitive function; it is also born from physical and emotional experience. In yoga, each event leaves its impression behind. The body retains the memory of everything it undergoes, an idea that is increasingly being confirmed by Western medical science. We now know, for example, more about how 'muscle memory' works and that it can take a year for the body to recover from the trauma of surgery. The same thing occurs with emotional impressions. The heart retains the memory of all our emotions, both positive and negative.

This huge store of mental, physical and emotional memories can lead to feelings of heaviness and overwhelm. The past is a trap if we are unable to escape its legacy. So many people I talk to are struggling to break out of patterns of behaviour so deeply ingrained that they feel inescapable.

But memory is not just an unchanging store of material, like some sort of internal archive. It's a process. We can work with memory as we can with imagination, learning to let go of what doesn't serve us and lay down new habits, new memories and experiences that support us. Just as you cannot create beneficial change without being able to imagine what it looks like, you can't create it without the workhorse of memory. Memory allows us to learn, to try something different from what we did last time, to set intentions and create new patterns.

This is a challenge for many of us. Releasing old memory, especially if it's emotionally painful, doesn't come easily. We struggle to allow the flow of feeling to pass through us and we end up with layers and layers of unreleased emotion, clogging up our organism. It's crucial to work on this. None of us can feel comfortable or stable if we're lugging a lifetime of baggage.

With practice, we eventually develop the capacity to distinguish between memories that we can work with and those we can't. Some emotional memories are so potent that eradicating them is impossible. In this context, the success comes from being able to keep an eye on your habitual feelings of mistrust, for example, without feeding them so that they become heavier.

Once we begin to shed the burden of memory, we are lighter

on our feet and the way forward feels easier. We are more aware of how our past affects our present and shapes our future. They intertwine in a complex dance that might be prone to missteps but is also beautiful and expressive. Memory is our mind dancing through time.

> *Explore an experience you've had, and discover what you've retained of it. What aspects of that memory you've held on to support you? Memory is necessary – but also a great polluter – are there any misunderstandings in that memory too? How does the memory link with part of your behaviour?*

Group 5: How can we develop the yoga mindset?

So, we're aiming to develop our aware mindset and spend less of our time and energy stuck in fighting or fretting. How do we go about it? How can we begin to get comfortable with sitting in the middle of chaos? There are a number of specific techniques given elsewhere in the *Yoga Sūtra*, such as physical practice (*āsana* or postures) breathing practice (*prāṇāyāma*), mantras and visualizations. We will begin to examine those in the next chapter. But first I want to look in detail at this section of the *Yoga Sūtra*, where it talks in general terms about how to cultivate a yoga mindset. Only by using the capacities that you have right now, in this moment, can you begin to cultivate this awareness – and that process of cultivation is in itself yoga practice.

I know you might be itching to hear about practical strategies and exercises, but long experience has shown me that it is counterproductive to jump into a programme of exercises before our mind is ready. Unless we first begin to clear up our perception of reality, including our own mental reality, we will take our bad habits straight into our yoga practice and this can exaggerate them. That's why it's so important to have grasped that yoga is a mindset, one among many, before we leap into yoga, either as a physical practice, as breathwork or as meditation. The life-changing magic happens when we can bring all these components together, and that can't be rushed.

Yoga practice = learning to sit at the centre of the storm (I.12)

Sometimes life feels like a tornado. We grab anything that might help us stay upright, even if it crumbles beneath our touch and leaves us dangerously exposed. We're so focused on clinging to these unreliable supports – our ex-partner, for example, or social media, drink, drugs or keeping an immaculate house – that we don't notice the serene spot we could aim for if only we detached, stumbled over and simply sat down.

Let's be honest, it's frightening to let go of your support – however unreliable – when you're being buffeted by life's storms. It isn't realistic to say that we 'just need to let go' of the thing, person or situation we depend on, without having something steadier to replace it. That's why so much of my work with clients is focused on swapping in positive and reliable habits for the old unhealthy and unreliable ones.

How can you tell the two apart? When you begin to practise, start with this simple aim: try to do more of what makes you feel better and less of what doesn't. Yoga occurs when there is a comfortable and stable link between you and whatever you're focused on, so we need to gradually loosen our attachment to objects (ideas, people, activities) that make us feel uncomfortable and unstable. We're better off deepening our attachment to objects and relationships that make us feel healthier and happier, such as our yoga practice, getting enough sleep, time outside in nature, positive social contact in real life etc.

One final word about the hierarchy of focus when you're doing this. Don't tell yourself you're giving up alcohol or your flaky ex, for example; instead tell yourself you're taking up breezy, hangover-free mornings, or running, or yoga. Concentrate on the new pattern of behaviour rather than the old one, and avoid any sense that you're rooting out something faulty or correcting a failure. This is not only much kinder to yourself; it's also more effective.

I once trained a woman called Priti to be a yoga teacher. Priti was such a great person. She ran a county court, so she was very senior and accomplished in her work, and she was also super generous and supportive to everyone on the course, not to mention being very glamorous and just generally lovely. Also, she smoked. Every time we took a break, Priti would nip out for a cigarette. She confided in me that she was desperate to stop smoking, but she'd tried many times and never managed to keep it up. This made her feel very ashamed. 'I've got to stop before I qualify to be a yoga teacher,' she told me. 'It would be ridiculous to be a yoga teacher who smokes.'

I told her straight out that I wasn't interested in this story of shame and smoking and guilt and failure. 'Stop trying to quit, Priti,' I told her. 'And stop telling yourself any kind of story about smoking. Just let the yoga do the work for you.'

Over the next few months, I noticed that there were fewer and fewer fag breaks. By the time the course ended, Priti hadn't smoked for nearly a year. She'd replaced that particular crumbling ledge with a much more reliable support. This one lay inside her, not outside: trust in herself to achieve her goals. Yoga itself is not the support; it's simply the way to discover that serene spot inside you that offers shelter from the storm. And the way to move from one attachment to another.

Can you imagine a stable behaviour that is so attractive to you that you want it more than whatever unhealthy or unhelpful support you're currently clinging to? How can you keep this same target and develop the experience despite anything that may come at you? How can it eventually become stronger?

Everyone and everything you encounter is your teacher (1.13)

Yoga can't be attained by reading something in a book (not even this one!), practising it once and – *bingo* – you've got a whole new attitude to life. Yoga is lifelong learning through a process of trial and error based on asking the questions that will allow you to see more clearly. Nobody else can do this work for you, because it is taking place inside your own mind and body. It has to be done over and over again because, while it isn't so hard to be comfortable and stable for a moment, we're aiming higher than that. We're aiming for (mostly) comfortable and (fairly) stable to be the norm. You are the only person round here who's going to come up with breakthrough insights that fit with *your* life and address *your* issues.

Learning yoga means practising it in daily life, but you're not practising in order to be 'good at it', you're practising in order to learn how it works for you. You practise by paying attention to every single interaction and every single moment. When you have a row with your mum, that's an opportunity to practise yoga. When you overhear a conversation about holidays at the school gate and everyone seems to have been somewhere fantastic and you feel envy and self-pity rising in you because you couldn't go away, in that moment those mums are your teachers and your feeling is an opportunity to learn.

Our yoga practice is not just a means to progress. It is also the effort we need to make in order to avoid defaulting to old behaviours. All of us will revert to type in situations that trigger us if we don't practise (and even if we do). Don't sweat your relapses; they're normal. Yoga is for life, and life will teach you yoga if you let it. Allow your practice to point you towards the wisdom you already contain.

Can you view your yoga practice as putting effort in and learning from your interactions in everyday life? Are you ready to stop looking to what's outside you to provide answers? Are you ready to allow yourself to find your own?

Stick at it and keep smiling (1.14)

I'm going to level with you: yoga is not a quick fix. In truth, I don't think there are any. If you need immediate relief from your backache, take a painkiller. If you want to understand why your backache occurred and what to do, practise yoga with an open heart and an inquiring mind. Yoga's like surfing, where success is directly related to hours on the board or fully involved in your daily life. You wouldn't expect to pick up a surfboard and immediately be able to perform Waikiki flips. You'd take it slowly and steadily while you built up your skill and your confidence. You'd fall off a lot and swallow a lot of water, but you'd hope to enjoy it along the way.

As with surfing (or any other demanding activity, from dancing a tango to speaking a foreign language), it might take years of practice before you can say that you've had success at yoga (which I define as feeling pretty comfortable and mostly stable, most of the time). But that hard-practised-for ease and calm will last you a lifetime. And this applies to your anxiety, your fatigue, your relationship with your mother, your relationship with *yourself*, just as much as it does to your backache.

Cultivating a positive and realistic attitude to your practice will make your learning easier and your growth that much greater. Don't judge yourself for lapses, just get back on track as soon as you can. It doesn't matter if you slow down, but try to stay in contact with the thread of your practice because, if you drop it, it's harder to pick it up again. And please, I implore you, wise up to your distraction techniques, objects of blame and excuses. I've heard them all in my time, from the relatively reasonable ('I've got a cold') to the really bonkers ('My legs are too long'). The one I hear more than any other is, of course, 'I haven't got time.' But as the Dalai Lama once remarked, 'I meditate for one hour in the morning, except for the days when I'm really busy. On those days I meditate for two hours.'

As TK said, 'If you can breathe, you can do yoga.' Just get on the mat.

> *What's your go-to excuse for not starting yoga, or doing your practice? How can you make the effort you put into it consistent over time? Is what you expect of yourself realistic or could you adapt?*

Yoga will unhook you from your triggers (1.15)

Fortunately, although yoga practice is definitely more tortoise than hare, more 'slow and steady wins the race' than a quick sprint for the finish line, you don't have to wait years to get to the good stuff. The rewards of yoga are not like the pot of gold at the end of the rainbow, always just out of reach; they're small daily wins, perhaps the gradual realization that you haven't had a bad day for a week or so. And they start coming within months, not years.

This *sūtra* tells us something about what I call the 'hookiness' of objects and how it diminishes with practice and new patterns. Fighting against desire never works; there is only ever one winner. How can you tell you're moving in a good direction with yoga? One way is to observe that you are reacting less to your triggers. The things that used to hook you in are beginning to lose their power over you. When I was beginning to practise yoga, my test case was crisps. God, I loved them. Couldn't get enough of them. If my stepdaughter put out a bowl of crisps on the kitchen counter I was powerless to resist.

Gradually, though, as the months went by and I reminded myself every time I popped into the kitchen that *I* was in charge, the crisps' level of hookiness for me went down and down. I still indulged occasionally, but it was with awareness rather than mindless grabbing. After a while I didn't even need to talk myself into control. It became automatic. This small change was a big thing for me. It felt good.

As we learn to detach from our cravings, question our fears and interrogate our actions, life feels easier. We are no longer triggered by the mention of our ex's name. We don't reach for chocolate cake whenever we're tired or sad. Detachment is not detaching from things but discovering that things detach from us on their own. We just don't need to fight internally because, as we practise, we feel better. We're on an upward cycle. Whatever unhealthy objects we're over-attached to, whether it's praise or wine or partners who put us down, we will need them less if we keep up with our new approaches. I find that so powerful.

How can we not fight against what we want to give up or let go of? How can we take a new approach that becomes a healthier habit for us? Can we maintain it so eventually it's we who are in charge and not the crisps?

Aim for progress, not 'perfection' (1.16)

Eventually, I didn't have to stand in front of that bowl and say to myself, 'Colin, you are stronger than the crisps.' The bowl didn't register. I literally felt nothing about it. It wasn't that the crisps themselves had become less hooky: it was that there was no longer a crisp-seeking hook inside me.

I can't say for certain that I will be immune to the lure of crisps for the rest of my life – that would be a fantasy fuelled by my ego, by desire and imagination. If I ever have a bad enough day, I might find myself scoffing giant packets of salt-and-vinegar. It feels unlikely, but it could happen, especially if I were to stop working on myself. My success with crisps didn't happen because I attained some sort of 'yogi perfection', since I remain subject to the push and pull of attachment and desire, as we all do. My success happened because I practised. And even if that success were one day reversed, it still happened, and I could make it happen again.

This is a really important *sūtra*. It says: you do not need to be perfect, either at yoga or in life. The aim of yoga is not to suppress your natural desires and attachments, or to eliminate all mistakes. Misunderstanding, as we've already seen, is by far the most common mental activity. Attachment is a normal part of being human. In fact, it is essential to your continued existence, since the subtle consciousness within us is fundamentally attached to the body that is its vehicle. I do not aspire to non-attachment. In practical terms, there's no such thing.

So, you're not aiming for complete non-attachment, or any other form of 'perfection', because it doesn't exist. Perfection is a category error. Initially, just aim for a little more clarity and self-knowledge, day by day. Gradually, you will realize that, though you still feel pain or irritation, the things that used to trigger you no longer drive you crazy.

Ask yourself, 'What's the best I can do here?' If you are a cancer survivor, for example, you may never be able to completely release your fear that the cancer will return. But if you can drive past the hospital where you had chemo without having an anxiety attack, that's progress. If you can accompany a friend there for treatment and sit by their side, that's a triumph. There is no longer a hook inside you. You are now in charge.

How does not being perfect sit with you? Can it be empowering to embrace the quirkiness of who you are? Realistically, what is the best you can do?

Don't get bogged down in the detail (1.17)

Life is like a game of snakes and ladders. You won't get to the end without having slid down a few snakes, so it's not worth getting hung up on any particular serpent.

This *sūtra* is all about the necessity of seeing the bigger picture and dialling down the drama that lurks in the details. Many of us are addicted to drama. We find ourselves getting swept away in a storm of emotion over something that we suspect (or even know, deep down) is not the main issue. The drama is a distraction that takes our energy in an unhelpful direction and risks escalating conflict.

So, when you feel yourself becoming agitated, or begin to

uncover turbulence through your practice, try to resist being caught up in it. This is hard. It takes practice. But try to notice what's coming up. Observe it. Remember that being able to see reality as it is, rather than denying it or misunderstanding it, is fundamental to making progress. You need to see more clearly, even if that makes you feel temporarily uncomfortable with what it is you're seeing.

In yoga we work slowly and thoughtfully from a starting point that reflects our clearest understanding of a situation as it truly is, not what we would like it to be or what we fear it will become. From there, we shuffle forward. This may not sound exciting or glamorous, but shuffling is sustainable and, if you keep it up, it can take you a long way.

Try to deal with the big stuff before you get into detail. I always suggest to people that they will feel better faster if they stop fussing over scraps of nuance (the 'he said this' and 'she said that' and 'that means I'm right!') and instead concentrate on the bigger picture of whether life is feeling better or worse overall. That is the only way to avoid falling into traps and relying on supports that crumble beneath our feet. It's the only way to live an authentic life.

Deeper self-knowledge and awareness is your lifelong aim. As your practice takes you closer to clear perception, you will experience many benefits. As your ego's needs diminish, you will find freedom, calm, strength and ease of body, mind and heart. You can exchange the appearance of enlightenment – what I call the fake 'light and love effect' – for a life that is consistently rich in reward and purpose. But only if you refuse to sweat every single snake.

Do you have a tendency to look for shortcuts? How can you replace this with a longer-term vision of what's possible? What steps could you put in place so there is a good order in where you want to go?

Group 6: Adjust and adapt

Context is everything (3.6)

This single *sūtra* – the only one in the book taken from outside the first two chapters of the *Yoga Sūtra* – is so crucial. It's about change, difference, diversity and the power that comes from being flexible enough to adapt to them.

We are all different, and yet many of us look instinctively for commonalities when we're relating to other people. We often seek the reassurance of concluding that, on some level, we're all the same, which can make us blind to the wonderful ways in which we are different. It's easy to overlook that we all perceive the world according to our specific background and the rules we've put in place, which are dependent on our context. This *sūtra* suggests that we might see more clearly and relate more successfully if we were to acknowledge, accept and celebrate difference. Such an approach makes me think of the way harmonies emerge in music when we play different notes that complement one another.

And just as there is infinite diversity between people, there is also huge diversity within ourselves. We are all many different people, constantly changing according to the shifts in our environment.

Change presents challenges. It can be hard to acknowledge that something that previously worked for us, no longer does. Maybe we used to be able to eat whatever we liked: cheese, chocolate, crisps, yet we never put weight on. So it comes as a genuine shock when we realize that we can't eat like that any more without feeling bloated and piling on pounds. Or we notice that the occasional glass of red wine that we've drunk for years now brings us out in a burning flush. 'Why is this happening?' we demand to know. 'I've been doing this for thirty years!' The answer is always, quite simply, that something has changed, in either the object, our environment, or us. With food it's very often to do with ageing, which sounds obvious, but it's amazing how many of us are so attached to our sense of ourselves as a skinny person, or a young person, or – OK – a *young at heart* person, that we can't see what our body is telling us.

This *sūtra* reminds us that we need to link with the right thing at the right level at the right time. Context is everything, in yoga as in life. It's important, for example, to get the level of your practice right for you. It's also important to remember that your right level might be different every day.

Do not lose sight of the fact that everything in life is relative. Changes in our environment and circumstances are constant so we need to be adaptable, in yoga as in everything. For example, sometimes you might need to let go of your rule that says you do thirty minutes of yoga a day, come what may. If you have a sick child and you haven't slept for three nights, what felt easy for you last week might now feel impossible. If circumstances change, let go of your plan and respond accordingly. Adjust your notions of success. Consider how much effort is the correct amount of effort for you *today*.

This isn't merely about giving yourself a break and taking things gently, important though that can be. On occasion you will need to make extra effort in order to pull yourself out of lethargy. Pay attention to your body, mind and heart and you will discover that you are not the same person today that you were yesterday. Your practice should adapt accordingly.

> *How can you tweak the aspect of your behaviour that is most troubling you at the moment? Rather than mentally searching for a solution, look around for an example of how somebody else has coped with the issue that's troubling you. Is there anything you can learn? How can you find the right level in your approach? Often, we keep doing the same things over and over again. Can you do something different?*

Group 7: What do you believe in?

Yoga is not a religion, but it does ask you to think about what you believe, who you trust and whom (or what) you defer to. It says we all need something to believe in. Can you identify the touchstones and authority figures in your life? Perhaps it's your boss or your partner, your friends or parents? The government? God? Do you defer to these authorities or compare yourself to them, rather than trusting your judgement and valuing your own experience?

Many of us hold unexamined beliefs about the world and our place in it that have been shaped by old stories, whether personal, religious or cultural. This can provide incredible support and strength; it can also lead us to duck our responsibilities and give away our power.

The *Yoga Sūtra* asks us to check in with these beliefs to ensure that they are a source of strength and courage. Are they intrinsic to us, or merely projections of what we've been told? Are they inherited, imposed or self-constructed? Beliefs can either empower or disempower us, so it's important to examine them with detachment and to check that they fit with us. It's rare to find that we need to reject completely what we used to believe in. Helpful adaptations will flourish if we invite them.

Our job is not only to understand what we believe and why but also what others believe about themselves and the world. All relationships are affected by the opinions, values and beliefs of those who participate in them. If we don't practise to understand where our friend, boyfriend, son, partner, neighbour, opponent is coming from, more conflict is the inevitable result.

Yoga does not require that we believe in yoga and nothing else. Whether it's our religious faith, our political views or our belief that we're a team player rather than a leader, these ideas are all absolutely valid and fully compatible with what we're learning in yoga. We also need to cultivate a core of belief in our own capabilities. We *can* figure out these (and many more) questions. There are no right or wrong answers, only greater clarity. Progress in yoga is built on taking responsibility for our own actions and trusting our own experiences to guide us. To live in this way is deeply empowering.

How can we have open-minded curiosity about another person's point of view? Can we accept that their reality and beliefs are different yet as valid and valuable as ours? Is it OK to agree to disagree?

Let go of comparison (1.18–19)

What is it about human beings' urge to compare themselves to others? We pretty much all do it. I'm beginning to think it's hard-wired behaviour, this need to rank ourselves in a pecking order. Maybe it's a primal thing? Wherever it came from, it's seriously unhelpful to our sense of self and our views on other people. It makes us feel bad about ourselves if we perceive that everyone else is doing better than us. It can make us into egotistical monsters if we decide we're the ones at the top of the tree. And who even gets to decide what counts as good, better or best?

This way of thinking is daft but powerful, and with the rise of social media it has a tighter grip on us than ever before. But while comparing ourselves to others might feel like a modern plague, it certainly isn't a new problem. The *Yoga Sūtra* discussed it thousands of years ago and I find what it has to say very comforting.

It tells us that, when it comes to success, there are three

kinds of people. The first are those irritating types who just seem to be good at everything they turn their hand to, from sport to relationships to exams to personal development. They are a tiny minority, but we tend to notice them because they're just so annoyingly good/good-looking/talented or whatever. The advice here is very clear: do not try to emulate these people. Their capacities are unusual and innate. You can't learn from them because they themselves did not have to learn to be this way, so they have nothing to teach. What a relief!

The second group comprises people who are fairly ordinary folk with regular struggles until they are set in a particular context. Then, suddenly, they shine. A musician may be feckless and selfish, for example, until they step on stage, where they pour out their soul with unbounded generosity. This group is a little larger than the first, but still small. Unless you also have their ability, don't try to take their pathway. You can't learn from them, either.

And then there's the rest of us. We need to work a bit harder to find our talent and our purpose, our contentment, stability and comfort, in pretty much every environment. We are the 'normal' ones, by which I mean that we are the vast majority. We need to cultivate faith that we're making progress, otherwise we lose motivation. We need to draw on the memory of previous successes when we're feeling down. We can't just breeze through life. We are also the fortunate ones, because we get to go on a journey. We get to grow.

Everyone is at a different stage on their path to yoga, as they are in life, and it's not a steady progress for any of us. Comparing yourself to somebody else leads only to frustration, discouragement and misery (or to unwarranted feelings of self-satisfaction). There may be a few exceptional people who seem to shoot straight to clarity – but, remember, they're a tiny minority.

Do yourself a favour and detach from watching anybody else's journey.

> *Are you someone who is good at everything you turn your hand to, or do you need to work at it? Does being in a particular environment work better for you in life? How can you reduce making comparisons with others to measure perceived success? Can you commit to cutting off from following other people's journeys in order to go on your own?*

Can you find a part of yourself that you believe in? (1.20)

We've seen that most of us need to work for the insights we uncover, just as we need to work for all our successes in life. This *sūtra* is speaking to us – those fortunate ones who are growing into success. It's a reminder that in order to keep growing we will need to stoke our faith, belief and conviction in ourselves and our trust in the process of exploration. It will transform our confidence. Yoga is a gradual discovery, not a revelation. It's all about our own process of trial and error. So if you experience a setback, for example, rather than reading it as proof that you're somehow failing, try to re-centre your faith in yourself and your trust that you can figure out what you need to do. Resist looking to somebody or something outside yourself for solutions to so-called problems. That so often leads to giving away our power and taking a turn that's wrong for us, rather than to the success we're seeking.

Faith in your ability to discover your own way might not come easily. Even once you've got your attention focused on your own journey as opposed to anybody else's, you still might find yourself getting dispirited because you can't meditate comfortably for twenty minutes. Then, a couple of months later, perhaps you realize you can sit for thirty minutes and you start to think you're the Buddha reincarnated.

Watch out for false beliefs attached to your highs and lows, in yoga and in life. One bad day – or even one bad year – does not make *you* bad. It's the same for a perfect headstand or a year of daily practice: they don't make you an enlightened yogi, or better than anybody else.

Remind yourself that you are doing what you can to make progress, and that's absolutely enough. Have faith that you are making your own unique way towards yoga and try to resist making somebody else responsible for your growth. That way you don't give away your power.

What is it you believe in? How does this give you strength or courage? How can the memory of that be reinforced to give more? What happens when you lose faith in yourself? How do you give away your power to someone or something else? Such observations can help prevent knocks to your confidence – turning them from disasters into huge opportunities.

Moonshots are powered by self-belief, not ego (1.21)

The stronger your faith, belief, trust, conviction and confidence, the more courage you have to draw on. The braver you are, the more you put yourself out there to learn. The more you learn, the more you trust yourself and the greater your stock of courage. These qualities are self-reinforcing. Bundled together they add up to self-belief, which is absolutely not the same as having a big ego. Self-belief is quiet, not shouty. It listens rather than drones on. It adapts. It is built on self-knowledge. And self-belief is rocket fuel for our yoga practice and our journey through life.

Keep the faith in yourself (and your practice) and everything will become easier. It takes time to build trust in your body's and mind's capabilities. That's fine. Ups and downs are fine. One day you'll feel a breakthrough into your core of fire that takes you to the next level.

Do you remember success or do you focus on failure? How can you prepare to access trusting relationships with yourself and others?

Success in life is directly linked to belief and effort (1.22)

Many of the outcomes we experience in life are determined by the restrictions we place around ourselves, or the expectations we set. I'm not talking magical thinking here but, by way of example, if you believe that you deserve a lasting relationship based on mutual respect and affection, you're much more likely to be in one than if you believe you're destined to get dumped by selfish narcissists over and over again. Your level of self-belief determines your choices, decisions and energy. It will shape your behaviours and lead you to a particular course of action. If you don't really believe in yourself or in the direction your life is taking, you won't put in much effort and you won't get very far.

Self-belief, or lack of it, is particularly important when we're moving from investigating and planning into doing mode. It's never a good idea to rush blindly into things, but once you've worked on your clarity, it's important to believe in yourself and let that fire you on. Otherwise, if your self-belief slips, the chaos of life will have you in its storm again. You can, of course, grope your way back to the calm centre as many times as you need to, but it's less exhausting if you can avoid too many slips. As far as possible, do only those things you believe in. And make sure you constantly foster the belief in yourself.

Are you putting effort into the right things? Which beliefs are you feeding with your energy and attention? Are you feeding courage or fear? If you don't know, or you're flailing around for the next step, is that a sign that your effort is taking you in the wrong direction?

Your preparation is complete

The foundations of your yoga practice are now in place. You've dug into how yoga understands the workings of mind. You've begun the lifelong process of asking yourself questions to deepen your self-knowledge. You're now ready to start the practical work of trying yoga out for yourself. This is a vulnerable moment but also an opportunity to check your self-awareness and self-belief. Are your beliefs and habits and patterns of behaviour becoming a little clearer to you? Do you trust in your own abilities to notice, assess and tweak your reality? How are you feeling? I really hope that as we reach the end of this chapter on the fundamentals of yoga as a mindset, you're curious and hungry for the next stage. It's time to start building on those foundations.

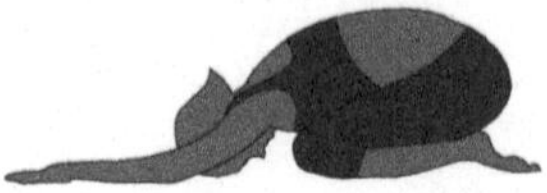

3. *Building Your Practice*

Yoga is like a machine for generating paradoxes. I sometimes feel I spend my whole life saying things like, 'On the one hand, yoga suggests this. But on the other hand it also shows us *that*.' This duality is fundamental to yoga philosophy. There's no such thing as an object that can be taken only one way. Our actions are always informed by our relationships, both looking inwards to ourselves and looking outwards to others. Yoga is all about the dualism of the world.

Perhaps there's an example of this in the way that I've been insisting that you can only learn yoga by *doing* it. Reading about it is not the same. I've also insisted that yoga requires us to prepare our minds as part of our practice, which means I've been insisting that you read about how to do that before you start doing exercises.

Actually, this is less of a paradox than we might initially think. After all, preparing the mind is not a passive process. It requires us to do far more than just read information. It's an active process of absorbing, filtering, asking ourselves those questions that have been running throughout the chapters, and reflecting on how our unique answers feed back into what we're learning about yoga. Laying those foundations is all part of the practice.

Now is the moment to introduce the discipline of active practice every day. It's time to ramp up a gear. This does not entail leaping into a complex programme of physical exercises or breathing work. It's enough to take perhaps ten minutes in the morning and ten minutes at night to use your body and breath to investigate your state of mind and review your actions and reactions.

From now on, at the end of each section there is a very simple exercise that is suitable for everyone, regardless of your level of experience. I encourage you to make these exercises part of your daily routine. You can use them in the morning or the evening. Experiment with them. Remember, there are no tests to pass and you can take everything at your own pace. Don't expect instant results or epiphanies. 'Practice' means doing something over and over again. The goal is not to do it 'perfectly', more to keep going until eventually each exercise becomes an integral part of your life.

Above all, try to pay attention to how you feel when you're practising. Everything from a twinge in your knee or a racing mind to a feeling of frustration will tell you something about yourself.

We will continue to work through the *Yoga Sūtra*, beginning to look in more detail at how to use tools and techniques to put into practice the ideas we've been reading about. The first tool we're looking at is breathwork.

Group 8: Let your breath teach you who you are

Watching the breath and then modifying it are central to all meditation practices, including yoga. *Prāṇāyāma*, or breathwork, is a tool for investigating our underlying patterns of behaviour and (eventually) changing them. When we do a breathing exercise we are very deliberately setting out to observe what is usually an automatic process. Then we modify it. We are now in charge of our breathing. We are laying down a different pattern of behaviour from the one that usually sweeps us along on autopilot. The learning here is potentially life-changing. If we can bring awareness to our breathing, which is usually invisible to us, we are creating a template for how to change other unconscious patterns of behaviour in our lives. *Prāṇāyāma* is the engine of change in yoga.

Conventional medicine also knows the power of breath to alter our mental and physiological state from one moment to another. How we breathe has a powerful effect on our nervous systems, which is why, for example, physiotherapists use breathwork to detoxify the body from a surge of adrenaline. Long, slow, deep breaths can be a fast-acting antidote to panic.

The longer-term uses of conscious breathing are less well understood by conventional healers, but yoga shows us that breathing reveals our moods and our beliefs; it helps us to build trust in our capabilities and can show us who we really are. Our breathing pattern is unique to each one of us, like a fingerprint or the way we walk, because the breath is the link between the subtle realm of your essential you-ness and the material realms of your body, feelings and thoughts. It's the channel through which you make contact with yourself and the mechanism for integrating all aspects of yourself. Breathing is simple and profound, like yoga itself. If you incorporate nothing else into your life, I hope you will take ten minutes to breathe consciously every day.

Bring consciousness to your breath and watch everything change (2.49)

This is another one of the great promises in the *Yoga Sūtra*. Even after years of study and practice, this line still makes me grin with delight every time I read it. It's a promise that we *can* change. We all have the capacity to replace our old patterns with new ones. Even better, we already possess and know everything necessary to make this change happen, because we can breathe and therefore we can change.

At its simplest, *prāṇāyāma* involves bringing awareness to your breath, and then altering it in some way. The outcome is to reduce the grip of those deep elements within us, such as anxiety or lethargy, that get in the way of our ability to meditate. So breathwork, like physical postures, is a tool for facing life head-on so that we can see more clearly. It takes practice to bring awareness to any automatic process, but the more we practise, the more capable we become of sitting down in the serene spot at the centre of our chaos.

I'm not saying that your habitual way of breathing is wrong, by the way. It's kept you alive so far, so it's obviously doing plenty right. But when you've mastered the basics of breathing, you'll have learned how to swap out an unconscious habit and replace it with a conscious one of your choosing. You'll have just graduated from Being in Charge 101.

This is so exciting in its implications that I want you to start right now. Turn to page 109 and read through the breathing exercise there. Now try it. Don't worry about doing it well or badly, just do it and see how it feels. Observe and reflect. I hope you feel a little flicker of excitement. Or maybe you feel calmer. Perhaps a bit intrigued. Now you're ready for more.

What was your experience of this breathing exercise? Can you observe how you felt before, during and after? What did you learn? Could you repeat this on a regular basis? Whenever you can be the observer of your own breath without having too much influence – this is the process of moving from unconscious breathing to breathing with awareness.

Discover a tool for profound, scalable change (2.50)

So, how do you practise *prāṇāyāma*? First, you pay attention to the framework of the breath, to its overall pattern. Do you breathe shallowly, short and fast? Do you frequently hold your breath when you're stressed or anxious? Do you breathe from belly to chest and back again, or hold your belly in and breathe from your upper body? You'll need to take some time to observe how you breathe in different contexts in order to build up a full picture. Try working with the exercise you've just tried as you do your job, as you speak, eat, drop off to sleep and whenever it occurs to you.

In general, a long smooth breath is healing for the nervous system and provides a solid platform for stability and comfort, but of course it's all relative, because every person has a different lung capacity and a different breathing style. Your long, smooth breath will be different from your partner's or grandmother's. There's no such thing as a minimum requirement for an exhalation or inhalation. The vast majority of us find that we could benefit from practising a longer, smoother breathing framework, but it's not a competition and there is no such thing as a standard breathing pattern.

Now that you're working on this exercise, and once you've got some awareness, you can begin to breathe in a specific and conscious way. The next step is to extend your out-breath, which you do by slowing down your exhalation in a sustainable way that you can maintain. If you find yourself either struggling for breath or holding your breath, draw back. You're overextending. After that, the next step will be to increase the length of your in-breath to meet the length of your out-breath. Then, the fourth step is to pause the breath at the end of the inhalation or exhalation, and to enjoy the space of the pause.

I always suggest that people start by focusing on the exhalation, because this is where we can learn the most. Exhaling places stress on the body. It makes us anxious because we are always, on some level, worried about where the next breath is coming from. Pauses between breaths are moments of vulnerability, and when we are vulnerable we have an opportunity to learn.

Retention, which is different from a pause, comes later. When you retain your breath you are creating a space inside you where, ideally, there should be no tension. This is not easy at first. It is intrinsically stressful to most of us to hold our breath. But gradually, with practice, you will start to understand something about how an action takes up space. Space inside your body; space inside your mind. You will begin to be able to hold something – in this case, your breath – without becoming tense, and to transition between holding and releasing smoothly rather than jerkily.

Gradually, you will learn how to combine all these ways of

breathing in patterns that feel restful or energizing to you. This practice can open the doorway to learning breathing techniques that affect your physiology, energy, psychology or spirituality. The overarching requirement for all this work is, over a number of breaths, to maintain a smooth, consistent and sustainable breathing pattern.

Start by developing your exhale (we have to empty beforehand to receive something new). Exhaling like a wave from abdomen to chest. Then develop your inhale to meet the exhale in length, smoothness and consistency. Breathing in smoothly from chest down to abdomen. Relish a pause without any tension at the end of the inhale and exhale – a point of freedom. Repeat this a number of times. With smoothness and consistency as the guide for your breath.

A portal into a new realm of awareness (2.51–53)

When we practise conscious breathing, we pass through a portal from the realm of mundane mental activities – all that ruminating, planning, desiring and fretting that we've talked about – into the realm of calm, of feeling alert and curious, engaged but not in need of anything. Here, our essential minds can be at peace: just watching the breath or the occasional passing thought. We might not stay in that realm for very long, but a few minutes can give us the opportunity to observe something unexpected. Even a few seconds can feel restorative.

To start with, most of us zap at warp speed back and forth through that portal. We're briefly at peace, calmly engaged and curious about what comes next. Then we remember that we were supposed to call our sister before we pick the kids up and, zap, we're back in the land of obligations and insecurities.

None of this back and forth matters once you've experienced the sheer joyous possibility of contact with the essence of you-ness, however fleetingly. The *Yoga Sūtra* describes the feeling as like lifting the veil of darkness that obscures the inner light of your you-ness. This effect is one of three things that happen when we develop our breathing and duck through the portal into another realm.

The first is that on the other side of the door we see things from a different vantage point. When stuff comes up, as it inevitably will, we're able to view it from a new angle. Hence what Fiona (from our introduction) said to me after her first ten minutes of *prāṇāyāma*, about seeing her difficulties with her relative from a new perspective. This shift in point of view can be very powerful, and though it often doesn't last for long, especially when we're starting out, it can feel invigorating and inspiring enough to keep bringing us back to practise.

The second effect is the sensation of being in contact with something rich and powerful and authentic and peaceful that we experience when we've lifted the veil of heaviness from our pure minds. And the third effect is one of increasing detachment from objects – the entrance gate to meditation. So it's not merely that we're seeing things from a different angle; we are also more distant from them. We have a little bit of room to manoeuvre rather than being squished right up against our desire for a glass of wine, or envy of our sister or fear of not becoming a parent.

These three effects of *prāṇāyāma* do not occur in any set linear pattern when we begin to practise. They might come all together or in rapid succession or slowly and sporadically. But as we keep on with our practice, we can direct them a little more.

Begin to observe what comes up for you when you do your breathwork over a few days or weeks. How do you feel before, during and after? What feelings and sensations emerge? It will be different every time, but gradually, themes will emerge. This emergence of a pattern is positive because it shows that you are providing the necessary space for whatever it is that needs to come up. One piece of advice. If you have a difficult decision to make, wait until after a breathing practice.

Breathwork builds your inner personal power (2.54)

Yoga shows us that *āsana* will build our learning in the outer world, but we need *prāṇāyāma* as well if we want to build our power in the inner world. When I began to practise, I thought my breath was a neutral object for meditation – not particularly exciting or enlightening but good enough. Now I understand that it is the dynamic link between aspects of myself and between the inner world of my essential self and the outer world of objects, thoughts and feelings. The more I focus on my breath, the more its apparent simplicity reveals layers of complexity. My breath anchors me within reality and simultaneously sets me free to explore it.

It's helpful to remember that 'reality' describes the inner realm as well as the outer one. It's not that only the world of objects, thoughts and feelings is real, while our inner world is mystical. They are two realms of the same reality. It's also important to understand that each of us can only be fully present in one realm at a time. If we end up straddling the two realms, that can weaken our effectiveness in both. You can't meditate and look after your two-year-old at the same time, which may sound obvious but its implications are important to remember. It's better to be 100 per cent aware in your outer world and then aim to transition smoothly to 100 per cent awareness in your inner world, than to try to dial down conflict in your outer world and pass through the portal to the inner world of meditative awareness, all at the same time. These realms are distinct, and our job is to get good at moving with grace between them.

This *sūtra* explores the idea that once we've passed through the portal to experience our own meditative mind, our essential self is changed by that contact. This inner change can lead to change in our outer world of speech and behaviour. We can become the agent with the power over how we link up with objects, rather than the other way around. The phenomenon is called *pratyāharā* (pronounced prat-yah-hah-ra), which means 'opposite food', and it is key to mastering cravings, transforming relationships and eventually living in freedom.

Before we can divert a troublesome stream, we first need to dig another channel in a good direction. The stream must flow into that new channel first, only then can we cut off the original that causes a problem. This is the wisdom of pratyāharā. *Recall an issue you are dealing with. How can you create a focus that is more positive and less harmful than the problem? Can you sustain it for time so that another channel is dug? Only then can you cut or create a dam to block the flow of the original issue.*

You are now in charge of your world (2.55)

The consequence of *pratyāharā* is that we are able to be the director of our senses and our self-expression. Each one of us has a particular susceptibility to certain sensory inputs, and we tend to over-rely on certain forms of expression. Many of us are highly visual people, for example, and find it hard not to be drawn by and crave beautiful objects. Others are particularly hooked by tastes, or the pleasures of touch.

As with the sensory inputs, so with the expressive outputs. Yoga identifies five of them: verbal communication, grasping things with hands, defecating, sexual pleasure and moving the body in space. And in combination these are the five basic ways we respond to stimulation and act in the world. So, for example, some of us have to talk everything over after a fight with our partner, others of us want to move away and be alone. Some of us have make-up sex.

Whatever our particular preferences, with regular practice of *prāṇāyāma* we gradually grow strong enough in our inner world to take charge of our hooks and habits. Rather than being slaves to ice cream, weak at the knees over the latest designer fashion or obsessed with sex, we are powerful enough to take charge of our sensory pulls, and to control our reactions to them.

Which sense do you rely on the most? Which sense is the one that leads you astray? Can you identify a particular way of reacting to circumstance that you perhaps over-rely on? How can you learn from your mistakes each time?

Eventually, for example, after I'd put in enough time on my mat, I no longer had to battle my desire to eat endless packets of crisps. There was simply no desire left. The hookiness had left the crisps and there was no corresponding hook left in me. Rather than the power lying in the object in the outer world, it had been transferred to me, and to my essential inner world. I didn't need to grasp those damn crisps. I could literally just move away instead.

As with sensory mind, so with the other seeds of difficulty that can take hold within us: ego and fear and aversion and desire. *Pratyāharā* transforms co-dependency into love. Instead of envying our sister we feel sincere pleasure on her behalf. Instead of banishing our anger with our father or suppressing our fear of failure, we welcome it in. Something has flipped and we no longer have to struggle to do the right thing. Sounds blissful? It kind of is.

An exercise to explore the power of your breath

1. Lie down so that you are comfortable, and place both hands lightly on your abdomen. Take your tongue softly to the roof of your mouth behind your teeth, and relax your jaw. Close your eyes. Feel the whole of the back of your body connecting with the ground. Now, as you inhale through your nose, take your breath in so it's smooth and consistent and your abdomen expands beneath your hands. As you exhale through your nose, again keep the breath smooth and consistent, looking not to overextend your breath in a forced way, as your abdomen sinks down beneath your hands. Keep your awareness on the contact between your hands and abdomen, between the back of your body and the ground. Repeat ten times.
2. Now bring your hands to your ribs. As you inhale through your nose, feel your ribs rise and your abdomen expand. Keeping the same consistency and smoothness, without any force, notice the abdomen and then ribs moving in as you breathe out through your nose. Maintain awareness of your hands on your body and your body on the ground. Repeat ten times.

3. Then, place one hand on your chest and the other on your abdomen. Keeping your eyes closed and your tongue in contact with the roof of your mouth, breathe in through your nose slowly, feeling your chest expand, ribs move out and your abdomen expand. This motion is almost like a wave that starts at the top of your body and makes its way down to the bottom. Then, as you breathe out, feel that wave pass from the lower abdomen back up through you. Use your awareness of the movement of the breath to explore inside your body while keeping an awareness of your hands on your body and the feeling of your body on the ground at the same time. Put effort in not to lose yourself in the practice but maintain your inner and outer awareness at the same time. Repeat ten times.

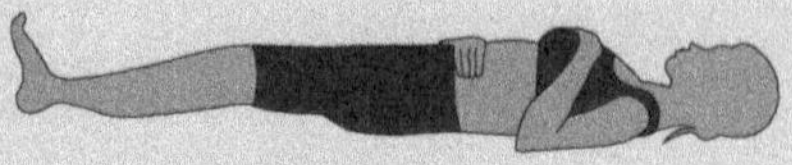

Once you're comfortable with the exercise above you could try the following variations.

An exercise for extending the length of the breath and incorporating pauses

1. Begin from the same position, lying on the floor with your eyes closed, your tongue on the roof of your mouth and your hands on your abdomen.

2. Inhale through your nose while mentally counting slowly to four and then pause ever so slightly before you begin your exhale through your nose. Again, count four as you exhale and then pause for a moment before you start your next inhale. It's really important to note that a pause is not the same as holding your breath. It's more like that moment when you're on a swing in the park, swinging back and forth and you're right at the top of the movement and seem to hang for a fraction of a second before dropping back down again. Same thing here: you're breathing in for a count of four, pausing and then breathing out for a count of four, pausing and then breathing again.
3. Repeat each of your long mentally counted breaths four more times. Then take a rest. You may want to repeat this again or increase the number of breaths.
4. As you get more practised you can attempt mentally counting for five on the inhale and five on the exhale. Then six, and seven and so on. It might take days or weeks to feel comfortable with these longer breaths. That's fine.

An exercise for letting go of counting while you breathe

1. Begin from the same position, lying on the floor with eyes closed and hands on your abdomen.
2. You're going to experiment with feeling your breath rather than counting it. You will naturally be aware of

when you're running out of breath, and now that you've practised extending and slowing and smoothing your breath, you have even greater awareness. So, rather than counting to four or five, use your voice to keep your mind focused and just feel the breath enter and leave your body as you repeat a simple sound. It can be voiced either internally or softly aloud on your exhale. You can use any sound or word that is meaningful to you. It could be as simple as the letter A, spoken long like Aaaaaaa, which I like because as the first letter of the alphabet, it symbolizes a new start.

3. Consider this an experiment that will build your sense of faith in yourself and your freedom. There are no rules apart from keeping the focus on breathing smoothly in a sustainable way.

Group 9: Step into your power

It is a truism that any action we take, including everything we think or say, post online, read, consume or choose, will have consequences. Yet we are very often surprised by those consequences when they show up. We struggle to anticipate what they might be. Worse, we forget that there is no such thing as consequence-free action. Everything we do lands somewhere in the world; it lands with other people and within ourselves. Our actions spark a chain of action and reaction that leads to a particular outcome. That might be positive – perhaps our action allows us to detach from heaviness or pain – or negative – our action might cause suffering by strengthening our attachment to unhelpful objects or habits.

The word 'suffering' sounds a bit melodramatic but, for me, it isn't confined to severe pain or the anguish provoked by tragic events. I understand it as a persistent feeling of discomfort, whether physical, mental or emotional. It's your dodgy knee or your weekly migraine. It's also your gut feeling that something isn't right in a particular relationship. It's the constriction of your heart that makes you tense and defensive rather then open and generous.

Suffering can be everyday, but 'everyday suffering' doesn't refer to every little twinge or any dip below 'happy'. Happiness is always a temporary state of mind just as feeling sad or bad occasionally is inevitable. But if your feellings of discomfort are persistent and distressing, please know that you can do something about them. This inspiring group of *sūtra* is full of fantastically crunchy but satisfying life lessons. It shows us how to separate what we can change from what we can't, focus on what's under our control rather than what isn't, and reduce those behaviours that lead to us feeling worse.

From now on, use the exercises to examine how you interact with people. Try to bring awareness to chains of action and reaction. Ask yourself questions about your motivation and expectations. Look to identify whether a particular action led to greater stability and comfort or more feelings of insecurity and discomfort.

Get beyond first impressions (2.12)

When we begin to investigate our motivations and feelings, we frequently get held up at the first layer of understanding. We notice, for example, that we snapped at our sister not *just* because she was being lazy about family commitments but also because we were already annoyed with her after an earlier conversation. That conversation, we can see, stirred up feelings of envy, which made us hostile to her when the discussion turned to something else: the question of whose turn it was to host Christmas.

This is a very useful realization. We often don't want to own up to envy, anger or resentment. So when we notice this motivation and connect it with an action, we are doing great work. But there is a difference between an impression and a consequence. The impression is the surface trace we notice on first glance. In this case, we notice our envy and connect it to snapping at our sister and her retaliating. But when actions are motivated by *kleśa* the reactions they trigger are similarly infused with *kleśa*. They leave more than surface traces; they can have deep and lasting consequences.

For example, our initial action in snapping at our sister was motivated by envy at her new job. Her retaliation returned the hostility and laced it with resentment for the fact that we're never pleased for her. Both of us dredge up the memory of all the times we've envied or resented one another in the past, and the situation escalates into a full-blown row. We then ignore each other for two weeks. Both of us feel we're drifting apart. We may feel sad about that, but project it as anger. Suddenly Christmas is a war zone and the whole family's wading in. Everything has escalated because we didn't do the necessary work to anticipate and take responsibility for the consequences of our initial envious feeling.

What would such work look like? It would start with a reminder to ourselves not to be satisfied with superficial thinking. There are many ways to avoid engagement with our own minds. We can reject ideas and emotions that make us uncomfortable: throw them out and away. We can repress them by pushing them down within ourselves. We can congratulate ourselves for figuring something out and then pop it back on the mental shelf and decide we don't need to look at it again.

One of the toxic ways that we get stuck at surface level is through making excuses for ourselves and casting blame on to others. Another way is through feeling guilt and shame, which makes us want to punish ourselves. If, for example, we decide that the envy we felt and the cross words we spoke were actually caused by our sister's insensitivity when she told us about her job, then we're blaming her and refusing to take responsibility for our own reactions. If, on the other hand, we decide we're a terrible person for having any negative feelings at all, we're taking on all the responsibility for the situation and punishing ourselves with feelings of guilt and shame.

More helpful would be for you to pause. Commit to going deeper. Ask where this envy comes from. Have you always felt inferior to your sister, ever since childhood? Or perhaps you consider yourself to be more successful than her, so this news bruises your ego. Or your identity is very invested in your job, but you are presently out of work and struggling to find a new position, so it's hard for you to be happy for her because you are scared for yourself.

Remember, you can't do this work of digging deeper when you're already having the row. You can do it either before or after the emotional interaction, but not during. When we're beginning to practise, most of us do it afterwards, once we've cooled off a bit. This is fine. Just don't leave it longer than a day or so to sit down and go deeper. Sift through what you said, what she said, how you felt, how she reacted and where that left you both, looking for more clues about what's really going on. Understanding your patterns of behaviour and taking responsibility for the consequences of your actions will make it far easier to fix old problems and avoid new ones. You'll be better placed to make a sincere and effective apology, which in turn will hopefully allow her to do the same. And next time one of you shares good news, you'll both be more self-aware about how you speak and listen, act and react.

What role or route do you tend to take in a difficult emotional situation? Do you blame others? Go into victim mode? Create excuses to justify? Use your vast array of distraction techniques? Curl up and ignore things? Or fall on your sword and take full responsibility? Most of us have an instinctive preference, and whatever it is, we over-rely on it.

Be brave enough to know your mind (2.13)

I generally don't do scare tactics; they're not very yoga. That said, I don't do reassuring platitudes either. The *Yoga Sūtra* stresses over and over again that every intention comes from either an openness of heart or a tight constriction of heart. Every action we do triggers a reaction, and where actions originate in the tightness that comes of *kleśa*, their consequences can be toxic. So I do point out to people that if they want to create positive change they can't be lazy and they can't fall back on avoidance, blame, shame or any other superficial and negative excuse.

We all have such safety behaviours. They are the tactics we adopt when we're feeling scared, nervous, uncomfortable and lacking the courage we need to commit to doing our work and taking responsibility for our actions. Safety behaviours are normal, but we can't move into the frame of mind where great change can happen until we get more practised at steering away from them.

This *sūtra* reminds us that, without the clarity of understanding that comes only from pushing beyond safety behaviours and first impressions, you'll be taking decisions based on incorrect or insufficient information. You'll be reacting from a tightness of heart. Problems will inevitably follow. It really is worth practising to go deeper, with more honesty and more detachment from shame, blame, anger or resentment.

The practice of yoga is the movement towards a clarity of understanding that has integrated all relevant knowledge. The rewards are less heartbreak and more joy. These are the fruits of long and patient practice, honestly owning what we find when we sit and meditate, admitting when we've got things wrong and making sincere efforts to do better. There's no short cut to acquiring this knowledge, but there's no alternative if we want to spend more time on the other side of the portal, in the freedom of our essential being.

> *Recall a situation that left a bad aftertaste – it didn't quite sit right with you. Identify which* kleśa *were involved that gave the quality of the experience you felt? How long did the effect of this experience last for?*

Same old crap, or something different? (2.14)

Every outcome, big or small, depends on your intention. Good comes from good and bad comes from bad. This is the basic principle of karma, or 'the golden rule', which crops up again and again in different world philosophies and religions. Think, for example, of the expression 'You reap what you sow.' Most of us understand that if we treat the world with hostility it will repay us in kind, whereas if we act from a place of empathy and generosity, we make it easier for other people to treat us in the same way. It doesn't guarantee that they will, sadly, and it's natural to struggle to trust people if our trust has been abused. But in the end we must learn to trust again if we want to experience joy and love.

So our motivation for our actions really determines how events play out for us. Get used to asking yourself honest questions about your desires and intentions. Are you gratifying your own ego and propping up your identity at the expense of other people? Or are you acting from a generous impulse to benefit others as much as yourself? If you consistently choose to act in ways that serve your own needs or desires and damage or disregard other people's, you are perpetuating negative chains of action and reaction. Sow selfishness, contempt, short-term gratification, ducking out of a challenge for the sake of a quiet life, and you will reap those results in turn. Sow consideration, generosity, giving people the benefit of the doubt and doing the right thing and you will reap all those instead.

This sounds clear enough, but even the most elegantly simple wisdom can get mangled out there in the real world. The 'do as you would be done by' concept is subject to all the usual human errors. If your intentions were good, for example, but somebody misinterpreted you, what then? I would say, just try to avoid blame or shame and clear things up through the most honest conversation you can have.

What if you suspect somebody else's intentions of being rooted in *kleśa*? How should you react to their action? Getting angry won't help, but you don't have to sit back and simply accept their actions either. You are allowed to meet them with calm, firm boundary-setting.

And if you're asking yourself how the hell you're supposed to know which place your intentions (or anybody else's) are coming from, I applaud your humility and say that you will know by watching the consequences of the action. Malign intentions manifest in malign results. If you practise clear-sighted observation after the event, you'll get better at picking up on the tell-tale signs when somebody's intention – or your own unconscious intention – was less than pure. This will allow you to react differently next time.

Unconscious intention can get the better of anybody. It happened to me during a phone call the other day. I didn't intend to be abrupt with the lady I was talking to about an admin matter, but I was tired and stressed and wanted to get the job finished. I could tell that I'd come over as aloof because her voice changed halfway through our conversation. She was suddenly short with me because she perceived that I'd been rude to her. It happens. Often we can apologize immediately, as I did, and both parties let it go. Sometimes, though, we have to dig deep to figure out what's going on. With effort, we can act from a place of good intentions and change our outcomes.

> *Consider the last time a conversation or situation didn't go the way you wanted it to. In hindsight, can you see anything in your intention that might have influenced the outcome and consequences? How can you make the right choice?*

'Change' is not another word for 'loss' (or 'opportunity') (2.15)

The volatility of nature is everywhere. It means that, really, there should be no surprises in this life. In reality, though, we often resist our own volatile nature and change in general. For example, something alters in our world (our grown-up children move out of the family home, say) but *we* don't change to reflect that reality. Or there's a naturally occurring change in us (ageing, for example) but we want to remain the same as we've always been. When we resist change in these ways we deny growth and development. If we embrace change as an ally, on the other hand, and use it as a spur to detach from the fleeting desires and demands of our ego, we give ourselves the opportunity to do better in the future. We open ourselves up to learning. We suffer less.

It's particularly important to use change as an opportunity to process our emotional pain. Not all change entails loss, but some of it certainly does. None of us is exempt from wanting more of something we can no longer have or mourning something or someone that has gone. When this happens we might suffer from disappointment, fear, envy, anger, resentment, despair. This is normal, and, as we will see later in the chapter, learning to accept these feelings is crucial to moving through them and releasing them.

This *sūtra* begins by acknowledging that change is typically perceived by human beings as a threat. We are, after all, hardwired constantly to assess our environment for danger, so if our context changes, we must (at least for a split second) assume that we are no longer safe. This threat might be perceived consciously or unconsciously, but either way it can make us feel sad, anxious, even crazy, because it uproots our points of reference. Yoga is precisely what will help us to regain our stability.

But the key message for me here is not so much the acknowledgement that change is tricky for all of us, consoling though that can be. It's the *sūtra*'s hint at the difference between how a sensitive mind and a meditative one approach change. A sensitive mind will perceive change and attach emotion to it, as well as interpretation and eventually a story or even a whole set of beliefs. The change ends up being 'good' or 'bad', a 'new beginning' or a 'disastrous ending'.

A meditative mind will perceive the change but, instead of holding it and classifying it, will simply acknowledge it and then set it aside. The meditative mind knows that, ultimately, the answer to whatever question we're asking ('Why did this happen?' 'Why has he left me?' 'Why can't I find the energy to do my dream job any more?' 'Why did she have to die?') is always the same: 'Because . . . change.'

This mantra is a reminder to me to meditate. To get some wisdom and remember that behind every specific answer to our questions about what has happened to us (even when those specific answers are both necessary and valuable) there is always this general explanation: everything changes. That includes us. When we sleep, meditate, think or feel, our minds alter. From day to day and week to week and moment to moment, the chaos is whirling inside us and outside us. All the more reason to sit down in the calm spot so we can pay proper attention.

Bring to mind a change that has occurred in your life. What emotions do you remember feeling? Stress? Fear? Avoidance? Denial? What rules did you put in place to protect yourself? Now consider the positive impact that particular change has had (or could have, even if it hasn't done so yet). It may be hard, but change is one of the only constants in our lives, so we must learn to trust that the eventual outcome will be manageable and even positive.

Problems are inevitable but suffering is not (2.16)

This may be my favourite line in the whole of the *Yoga Sūtra*. (Admittedly, I say that about a lot of lines.) It's a brilliant, powerful, empowering promise that says, 'Life doesn't have to be a nightmare. You *can* reduce your future suffering by changing the way you act and react to things, people, events right now . . .'

This is really the heart of what I want to tell you. Yoga can't promise that it will enable you to get through life without pain or difficulty, because pain and difficulty are fundamental elements of being alive. But yoga can show you how to handle that pain and reduce its negative consequences, how to tackle difficulties calmly and with clarity. Every time you practise yoga, you're teaching yourself how to suffer less the next time the shit hits the fan.

And, let's face it, shit-hit fans are always out there. Every single one of us is made miserable by something, but every single one of us can also learn to work through our misery and suffer less. The only way to do this is by taking charge. Refusing to be drawn into drama, sidestepping the pull of unhealthy habits. Analysing your part in toxic relationships and choosing to step away, without blame or shame. Above all, you reduce your suffering by realizing just how much power you have to make it bigger or smaller.

I have never forgotten an argument I had, years ago, with my partner at the time. We were going round our usual track of grievance and counter-grievance when I suddenly saw, very clearly, that I could prevent an enormous amount of unpleasant feeling for both of us if I just . . . sat down and listened to what was being said to me. Really listened, without interrupting or planning clever ways to score points. So I told them, 'I'm going to sit here and listen to you because you're right; I need to do that.'

It changed the whole feel of the conversation. We each still saw the situation differently, and we were still divided over what to do about it, but we were no longer fighting blindly, rational thought completely overpowered by our emotions in the moment. When that fight ended (and when the relationship subsequently ended), we knew one another and ourselves better than we would have done if I hadn't sat down in the middle of the storm. We were able to be more honest and kinder.

Some people mistake this sort of opening up for an admission of defeat. I see it as a way to step *into* your power. When you sit down to pay quiet attention you're not signing anything away, you're simply freeing yourself from the grip of emotion and from the tyranny of old stories or beliefs. You're averting future distress. We all have the power to do that.

The next time you feel a storm approaching, whether it's a difficult conversation with your partner or a tense family meeting, can you hold a single intention in your mind and your heart as you contemplate this challenge? The intention is very simple: when you are talking with the other person you will not draw any lines in the sand. You will not box in either yourself or the other person. This will be your open-hearted intention as you go into the conversation. The message is act now; you can prevent future issues.

Life is for exploring and enjoying (2.18)

I recognize that going anywhere near the meaning of life risks sounding like the set up of a joke, but *Yoga Sūtra*'s answer to the question of what life is *for* never fails to make me smile. This *sūtra* insists, quite simply, that you're here on Earth to maximize your enjoyment in being you. The most effective way to do that is to understand just how much freedom you have. Happiness is a by-product of living your best life and feeling free. It's not the goal.

Sure, there will always be burdens, responsibilities and struggles in life, but you can choose either to labour under them or to dial down their impact. Life can be lived as a series of either trials to endure or opportunities to detach and learn. If you opt for the latter, you minimize your suffering.

There is no higher calling than to step into your own freedom of mind and discover how comfortable it is to be yourself. (And, no, this has nothing to do with sensory pleasure or gratification of ego. I didn't need to say that by this stage, right?)

> *Going through your day today, can you completely involve yourself and be fully aware of each situation and its surroundings? As you move from one situation or set of surroundings to the next can you immediately adapt to do the same without carrying across anything from the previous one?*

Who are you, really? (2.19)

Most of us have a tendency to jump to conclusions. We crave answers to problems and love a good generalization. The way we tackle projects or gather knowledge is typically not by slowing down and looking more closely at specific detail but by building a grand theory from our own personal experience of what we consider to be correct. Needless to say, that usually gets us into trouble.

If we can detach from our fondness for the superficially convincing we can embrace a beautiful evolution in our understanding of everything in this world, from the general and unspecific towards the unique. As we learn to differentiate between objects, we discover what makes them truly themselves. There's a reason that we were all made to write those 'compare and contrast' essays in school. Asking how things are similar and how they are different is a fundamental way of classifying and interpreting what we see around us.

It can be helpful to work *with* rather than against this flow of understanding because it has such a powerful practical resonance. When we're planning a project such as a house move, for example, it rarely helps to make our initial requirements too specific because that risks limiting us to a plan that's rigid and unrealistic. If we were to decide at the outset that the only acceptable house is within five minutes' walk of a Tube station and a park and a good school and a pub that serves our favourite beer, then unless we have a very big budget, we might struggle to find somewhere to live. If, on the other hand, we start general and then let the plan unfold towards specifics, tweaking matters along the way, we will probably end up with many more options.

As with objects such as plans, so with ourselves. We are all on an evolutionary path towards discovery of the essential core of who we are. We start out with a full set of assumptions about ourselves and other people, perhaps thinking that we're much like everyone else (even as we crave validation for being exceptional) or believing ourselves to be superior or inferior. We see only generalizations and misunderstandings. But if we follow our path of meditation, we end up appreciating who we really are and working with that unique potential. We evolve from the generic to the specific and become who we truly are.

Next time you meet someone new, experiment with not coming to immediate conclusions or making assumptions about what or who you think they are. In conversation with them, let them speak, ask questions and see what comes to the surface.

Exercise to explore action, reaction and consequence

Your aim with this simple sequence of postures is to use them as a way to explore some of the key themes of our work. The movements themselves are not significant.

Firstly, I'd like you to be aware, while you do them, of the idea that there is a difference between your body, which is the medium for your exploration in this exercise, and the part of you that is in control and making decisions about how to move. Practise observing the way your body feels and the way your mind feels. This slight separation between the observing part of yourself and your body and mind (the material parts of you) allows you to practise disengagement and encourages you to pay attention to your actions and reactions to events.

Secondly, once you've established the distance to observe, practise observing the consequences of your actions. For example, if you are pushing too hard as you do these movements, you might feel some discomfort. If you do not make enough effort, you might not feel any effect. If you feel good after the sequence, you might notice your ego emerging to tell a story about how great you are at yoga. You get the idea. Every single action or reaction has consequences. It's our job to train ourselves to observe this and, without judging, decide whether they are the consequences we want, or not.

Repeat this sequence every morning for the next week. Do you notice any changes from one day to another? Are there emotions that arise often? Or do you start out feeling enthusiastic and finish the week feeling dispirited? Whatever comes up, remember not to attach meaning to any of it too quickly. The aim of the exercise is to practise your ability to notice what's going on. That's all. You don't need to know what anything means or have a plan for how to change it. Those stages evolve in their own time as your understanding of how you do things reveals more and more of how you interact with yourself, other people and the world.

Practice 1

Sequence I:

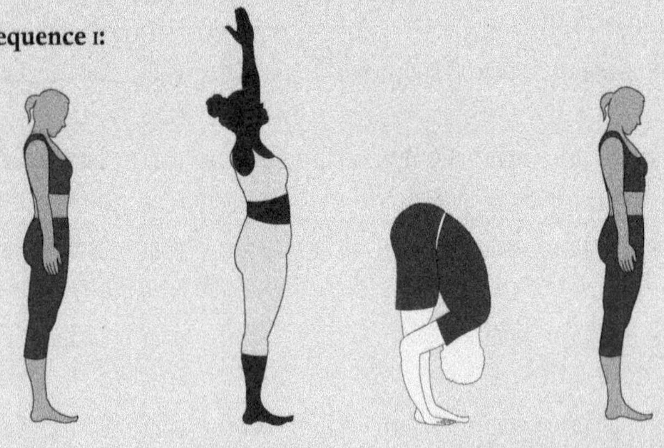

1. Come to stand, arms by your sides.
2. As you breathe in, move arms above head.
3. On your breath out, bend knees, fold forward. Take a breath here. Breathe in lift your chest, raise your arms, come back to stand. Rest your arms down.

Sequence II:

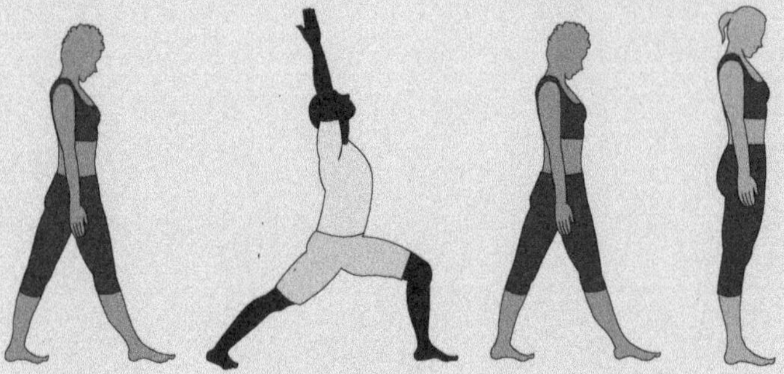

4. Turn one foot slightly out to the side, step the other foot forward. Take a breath here.
5. Breathe in, bend the front leg at the knee, raise the arms above your head. Take a breath here.
6. Breathing out, lower arms and straighten leg. Step back to bring both feet together. Repeat, taking the other foot forward.

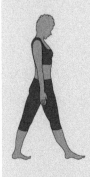

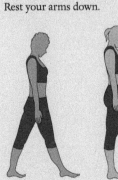

Practice 1

Sequence III:

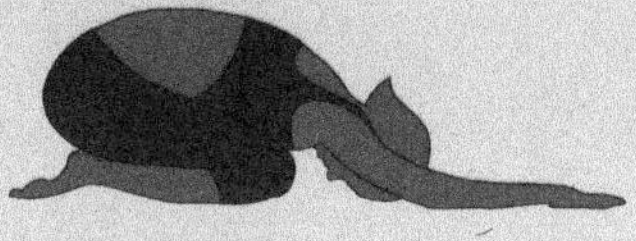

7. Lower your bottom back to your heels. Take a breath here.

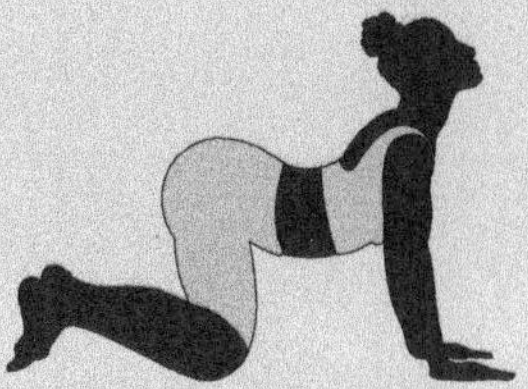

8. Breathe in, come forward to your hands and knees. Take a breath here.

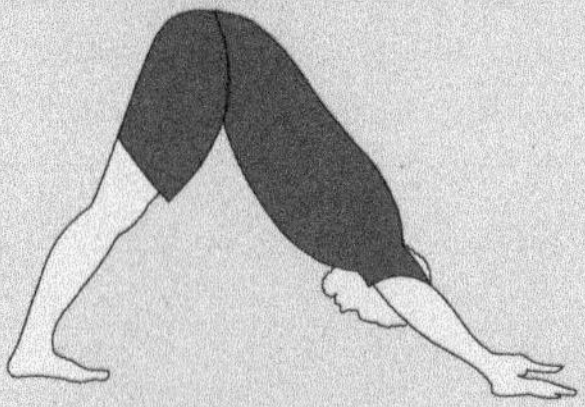

9. As you breathe out, lift your knees off the ground and raise your bottom into the air – keep your knees bent if you wish. Take a breath here. Lower both knees down on your next in-breath. Take a breath there.

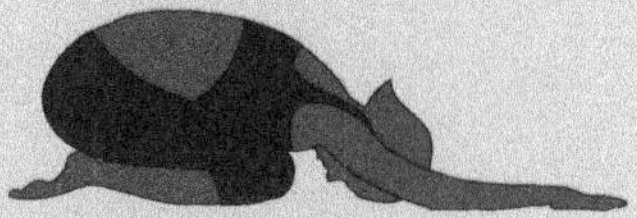

10. Breathe out to take your bottom back to heels. Take a breath.

    Repeat as many times as you feel is helpful.

Final pose:

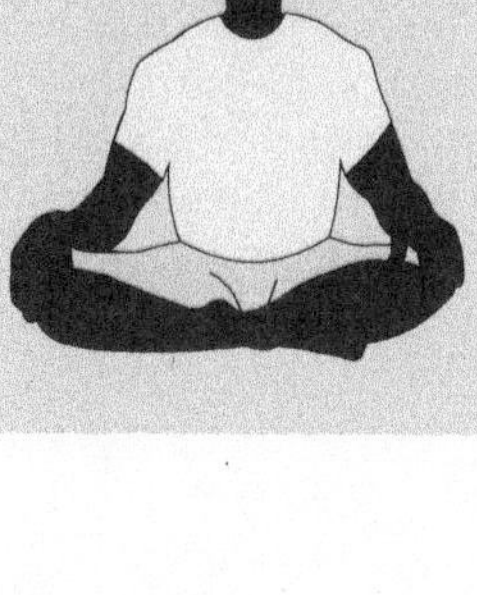

11. Then, come to sit in a comfortable position, feeling your body. Bring your attention to your breath, focus on keeping your inhale and exhale smooth and consistent.

Practice 2

Sequence I:

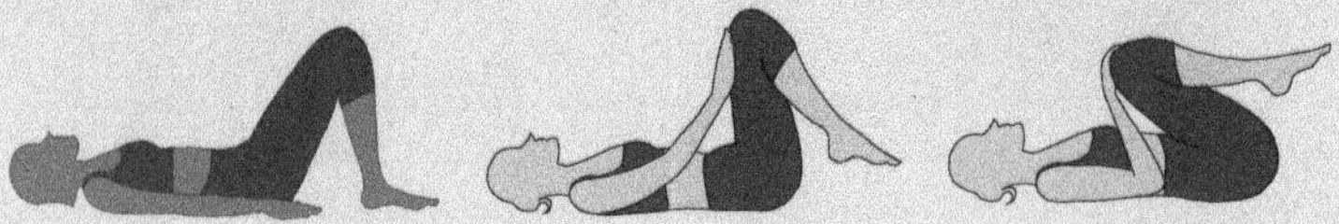

1. Lie on the floor, legs bent, arms by your sides. Slow your breathing down, make it smooth and consistent.
2. Lift your knees towards your chest, take a breath here. Then place your hands on your knees. Breathing in, guide the knees away from you. Breathing out bring your knees closer towards you. Repeat as many times as feels comfortable, moving slowly and steadily.

Sequence II:

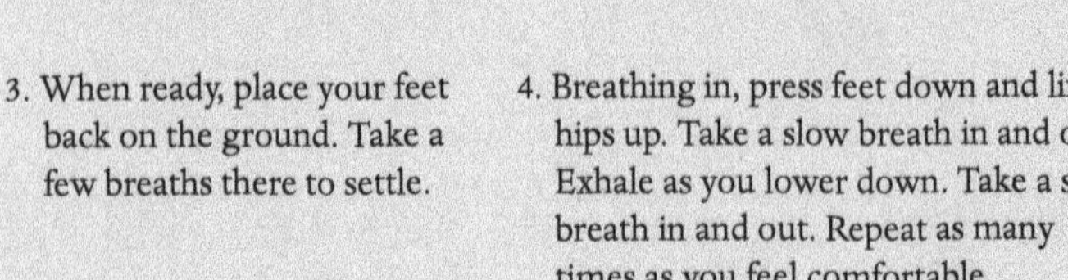

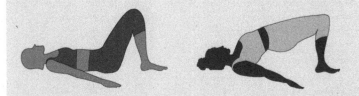

3. When ready, place your feet back on the ground. Take a few breaths there to settle.
4. Breathing in, press feet down and lift hips up. Take a slow breath in and out. Exhale as you lower down. Take a slow breath in and out. Repeat as many times as you feel comfortable.

Practice 2

Sequence III:

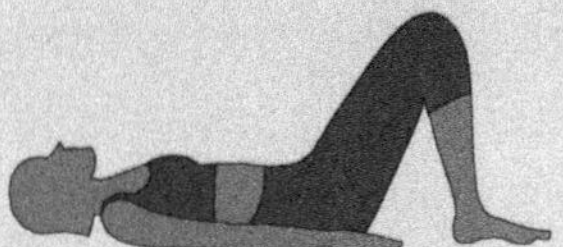

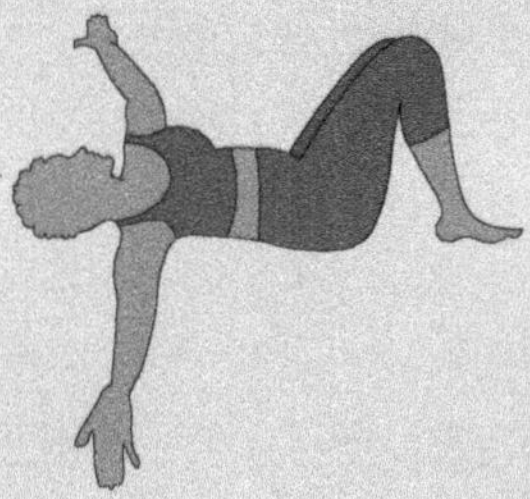

5. Take some breaths here with your feet on the ground. Back of your body on the ground.

6. Breathing in, slowly move your arms out to the side. Breathing out, carefully lower both knees to one side.

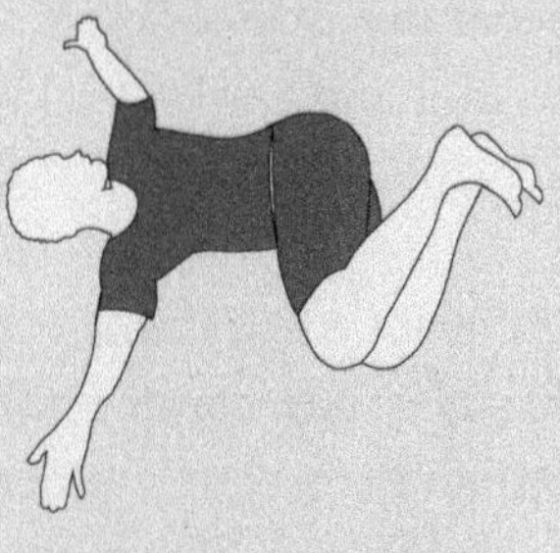

7. When you are ready, inhaling, slowly raise both knees back to the centre. Take a slow breath once there. Then lower both knees to the other side and repeat this sequence as many times as you feel comfortable.

Final pose:

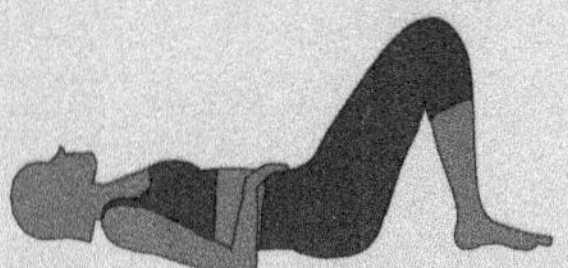

8. Finally, settle your body. Place your hands on your abdomen if that feels comfortable. Bring your attention to your breath, and the movement of your abdomen as you inhale and exhale. Take as many breaths as you feel comfortable.

Group 10: Freedom is a state of mind

We're all prone to getting lost in mindless thinking. It's easy to be distracted by worrying about an upcoming meeting or feeling bad about snapping at your toddler. We are prisoners of our attachments, over-involved with the things and people that surround us; far too over-involved with our emotions. When the essential part of our consciousness collapses into these swirling waters, we lose control and freedom. Yoga is the lifeline we can use to haul ourselves to a calmer place, one where we still feel our emotions and care about what matters to us but don't drown in the torrent of feelings and claims on our attention. We can resolve problems without becoming too distressed by them.

This group of *sūtra* investigates how to create space between your essential self and the mental activities and *kleśa* that throw a veil over it. It shows you how to separate yourself from conflicts and dramas, how to resist the pull and push of objects and people and respond nimbly to events in a way that feels right to *you*.

I want to reiterate that attachment is not a bad thing – quite the opposite – but we will live more stably and comfortably if we can loosen our attachments rather than cling harder to them. This is one of the ultimate goals of yoga. The more we practise it, the closer we come to uncovering our own individual purpose in life. Having a sense of our purpose allows us to feel safer and more secure, which makes our evolution so much easier. In a mutually reinforcing process, we both see more clearly and shine more brightly so that we can be seen as we truly are.

You have so much more agency than you know (2.20–21)

I meet a lot of people who feel powerless. Some of them have given up in the face of physical or mental suffering. Their pain is so great that they have no courage left. Others have given their power away through fear of change. Some are powerless in the face of their addiction. Some are struggling to see how they can break free of the stories they inherited from their family or the society they grew up in.

All these people are having a hard time and the pain they experience is real, but it's also made much worse by the story they are telling themselves about it. Every person who assures me that they can't do yoga until they're well, or they can't divorce their husband because of the children, is telling me a story to explain their decisions and actions. I have heard these stories before, but I have also heard their opposites. Some people say to me, 'I feel so awful: I'd better start practising again.' Or, 'I have to divorce my husband because of the kids.' There is no right or wrong here. There is only the weight of evidence, gradually stacking up, that some stories lead to more suffering and others to less.

I feel so much compassion for all these people. I listen and empathize and listen some more. Then I break the news that's contained in this *sūtra*: you have so much more agency than you know. There are so many different spaces available to you within your mind, and so many different stories you could tell with these raw materials. (The *Yoga Sūtra* puts this firmly but gently, by stressing that it is possible to be fully involved and yet not attached. I tend to be a bit more blunt.)

Your body and mind exist to serve your pure consciousness. How you use them is up to you. This *sūtra* says that every object (person/event/thought) in your life exists to serve the essential you-ness that is your pure consciousness. No matter whether you're struggling with mental health disorders or addiction, wrestling with life choices or just trying to stay calm as you drive home from work through heavy traffic, ultimately, you're in charge. Or you could be, if you practised.

Sometimes, of course, we find ourselves with very little control over our circumstances. You might be feeling powerless right now, and pretty irritated by me telling you that you're in charge. But whatever your context, life presents you with an opportunity to react to it. You have choices. If you react from a place of fear, desire, anger, ignorance, things will go worse for you. If you are able to clear those obstacles away and see more clearly and calmly, you can step into your power. What I want is for you to be fully conscious, to be as much yourself as possible.

The key is to practise loosening attachments and slowing down your emotional responses. Create and use that space between your clear mind and all the swirling chaos. Remember, once you've been sucked into the swirl of events, the lifeline of yoga will be temporarily out of reach. You can practise creating distance before or after an argument, for example, but not once you're in it (at least until you've clocked up a fair amount of practice). But even if you miss the first opportunity and the row breaks, there will be another moment – after the shouting and sulking stop – when the lifeline of yoga is yours to grasp again. You are not your anger; you are something else. Anger comes and goes but you remain. Understanding this difference is the key to freedom. Your life is your opportunity, the only one you will ever have. How can you do the best you can?

> *How can you be involved and active in your life but not too involved in all its passing dramas? How can we do the best we can in each situation and nothing more?*

Stop catastrophizing – your life is not a disaster (2.22)

Yoga shows us that all matter (our bodies, our minds, the queue in Aldi) has a purpose in relation to the non-material or subtle realm, which is made up of the pure essence of each individual being. Once a material object has served its purpose, it must change into some other form. If we are wise, we will recognize that and let it go.

This is not easy. So many of us freeze up in the face of reality's constant dance. We refuse to accept that things change, that people and outcomes and hopes and dreams slip away from us, despite all our planning and checking. Of course, change can be painful and life is full of loss, from the trivial to the enormous, but it's our refusal to process the sadness and anger that accompany these losses and then change our reactions to them that really compounds our suffering.

I encourage you to think of change as a transition from one state to another. Every one of these transitions offers us an opportunity either to put something down or drag it with us into the next moment. Some of these transitions are profoundly important. If you are coming out of a painful divorce, how many of your beliefs about love and relationships do you want to carry with you and how many would you do well to put down before you begin the next phase of your life?

But I'm not just talking about huge losses such as divorce or bereavement. Every interaction we have, every small worry or decision, can provoke negative feelings. Every day is made up of small transitions: shifts from one space, way of thinking or attitude to another. When you finish work or get back home from college, for example, you need to transition into your 'at home' mindset. You need to allow the other people around you to transition too, in recognition that you've arrived. There's a classic moment of tension between couples, especially if they have young children, where one partner gets home after a day away and the other wants to launch into conversation, or hand over responsibility for the kids and run off to their next activity. If you can give yourselves and each other space to live that change comfortably, tension can be avoided. To my mind, managing a moment of transition like this with awareness and serenity is at least as much yoga practice as any physical posture. The more we do this, the better we get at staying calm despite chaos.

I meet so many people who tell me that they are overwhelmed by work pressures, family commitments and the endless to-do list that is modern life, by their feelings about past choices or fears for the future. Most of us don't notice that feeling overwhelmed comes from being *over-involved* with every tiny detail of life's ebb and flow. We pour emotional energy into worrying, ruminating and checking on everything and everyone rather than practising gentle disengagement.

A high proportion of my conversations with clients begin with them telling me some variation on, 'Everything's a disaster.' I try to help them see that it really isn't. Even if they are having a truly terrible time, those particular circumstances will pass. And there are things they can do to help them pass more rapidly and prevent them from happening again.

Have you ever realized that you were caught up in the drama of a situation? I still get this sensation sometimes. When I moved house last year there were various tricky moments involving negotiations with estate agents, lawyers, surveyors, buyers, sellers and all *their* lawyers. At one point we thought we were going to lose the house we loved, which suddenly felt as if it would be a complete disaster rather than merely a shame. I was having so many tense conversations with so many people that I realized I'd spent thirty minutes scrolling e-mails and composing a justification of our position that nobody had even asked for. Once I'd noticed, I was able to stop, step away and breathe. Within a few minutes I could laugh at myself for getting so caught up in all the 'stress' that I'd lost sight of the fact that I was still in the very fortunate position of being able to buy a lovely house. I had turned a routine process into a huge 'poor me' drama by allowing myself to get over-involved with its every inevitable twist and turn.

Bottom line: don't let emotion take your power away. The moment any feeling comes up for you, remind yourself who's in charge. Every transition, even the most painful, is an opportunity for you to evolve – but only if you can disengage from over-involvement.

Can you identify a change occurring now in your life that you're either not engaging with, resisting or are over-involved with? Can you adapt from this one situation to another? How can we reduce the normal complication and make things simpler? When someone is speaking, can you listen even if you know what they are going to say?

Attachment can be a highway to self-knowledge (2.23)

Sometimes people form the idea that yoga and other Eastern philosophies are saying that attachments are 'bad', something that we ought to be able to let go of, or get past. This can feel like an attack on the emotional ties that bind us and make us resistant to the wisdom of these philosophies. As one lady put it to me, 'I don't want to let go of the people I love!'

You really don't have to. Nowhere in the *Yoga Sūtra* does it say that being attached to your loved ones is bad. But there is a difference between loving attachment and co-dependency, which illustrates something useful about the difference between grasping or clinging on one hand and gentle enveloping on the other.

As we've already seen, attachments are an essential and beneficial part of being human. They keep us safe and give us the opportunity to learn and to love. Without secure attachment a child cannot thrive, for example. Without a passion or purpose, life is dull. Attachments allow us to have interactions with other people, with ideas and aspects of ourselves, all of which facilitate our evolution.

Attachments can also get us into trouble, not least because they (like everything in the material realm) are always changing. Your relationships depend on your attachments to other people. Your sense of identity depends on what you value, what you choose, decide, etc. – all forms of attachment between you and an object. If these attachments are lightly held they are more adaptable to the inevitable volatility of nature. Rather than clasping your loved ones or your beloved aspects of your identity too tightly, it's better to envelop them with a softer embrace. This will allow you to suffer less and learn more through your interactions with other people and with aspects of yourself.

The most fundamental attachment is the one between our subtle consciousness – the 'essence of who we are' – and the material realm of our bodies, thoughts and emotions. Without our bodies our consciousness would have no vehicle, and life as we experience it would be impossible.

This strong link between our consciousness (what yoga calls *puruṣa*) and the material (*prakṛti*) is the greatest learning opportunity we will ever have. Once we become aware that there are two aspects to our being and that they need each other absolutely, we are in a good position to integrate them so that they can get on with their tasks as part of the team. It's a bit like the trusting teamwork in any healthy and happy life partnership, where both partners have each other's back. You need to have your own back in the relationship between the two sides of your self.

Investigate and embrace the intense attachments between your body, mind, heart (the material realm of *prakṛti*) and your essential being (*puruṣa*). This is not a simple thing to do, of course, but it's so empowering to try. And it will heighten your understanding and enjoyment of who you are, which is really our whole purpose in life.

> *Everything has a role in life and can bring something to you. Attachments are fundamental to life. Can you be OK with that? This means being OK with your attachments to things and to people.*

Learn to adjust your emotional perspective (2.24)

Sometimes people confess to me that they worry they will never learn to get a handle on their anger, or their grief or their fears. I always reassure them that this is not the case. Yoga is a tool for liberating yourself from the grip of whatever negative emotion you struggle with, but you have to practise. The key skill is your ability to recognize your own feelings faster, and then react to them in ways that head off problems. The better you get at this, the more easily you can steer away from hostility and error.

Every relationship, whether it's between aspects of yourself or with someone else, will go through highs and lows. Sometimes there is peace, sometimes conflict. It's hard to maintain perspective on these ups and downs and hard to preserve the necessary detachment from the emotional turbulence they produce. Often, the best we can do is hang on to the truth that every interaction is an opportunity: either for trouble or for learning. I just try to make sure there's more learning than trouble!

The problems of maintaining perspective and avoiding emotional over-involvement are, of course, closely linked. Human beings are deeply emotional creatures, which, on the one hand, makes life worth living but, on the other, can also feel troubling and frightening. We need to practise being brave and agile enough both to flow in tune with our emotions and to stand firmly back from them as necessary.

The first step is to get more comfortable with all feelings. We won't learn anything if we deny them by pretending they don't affect us or by putting on a mask and performing a more 'acceptable' version of them for other people's benefit. Second-guessing other people and faking our feelings will only ever make us less loving, more controlling and much more anxious.

We won't learn if we ignore our emotions, either, or if we

panic and run away from them or try to push them on to another person. All of these reactions will lead to trouble rather than learning.

Once we've mastered our first instincts to flee, or cover up, or deny, the next step is to find a good vantage point from which to consider our feelings. We're looking for the spot that grants maximum clarity and freedom of action. This also takes practice. Sometimes we can't see what's going on because we're too close to get the full picture. We can't act either, because we're squashed by the fast-moving dynamics of the situation. Sometimes the problem is that we're too far away to see anything at all. We've become so detached that we have neither clarity nor engagement. In either case, nothing's going to change and we're not going to learn. So, in yoga, we are constantly looking for the way to be involved but not over-involved. What do we need to take from an interaction with somebody who has annoyed or upset us? What do we need to leave behind? What should we integrate and what should we release?

The fact that you can't see something doesn't mean it's not there. Could you be open to reflecting on a situation that's caused you a problem? View the situation with you in the overall picture too. Examine whether you are too close and involved. Or perhaps you are too far away. Either will affect what you know and don't know.

Embrace not-knowing and feel the freedom (2.25)

We've seen already that, in yoga, the root of all our troubles is that we don't see clearly and we don't know or understand reality. Our perspective is clouded by fear, ego, desire – all the inevitable *kleśa* that get in our way. So we're always trying to reduce the impact of *kleśa* and increase our ability to assess reality clearly.

And yet . . . because this is not a perfect world and we are not perfectible creatures, we must embrace the fact that we will never attain 100 per cent clarity or 100 per cent correct understanding. We can aim to reduce our misunderstanding but we cannot hope to eliminate it. In fact, we must practise being comfortable with all that we don't know at the same time as we work gently to reduce it. (I hope you're getting comfortable with yoga's paradoxes, because they just keep coming!)

Last year I was working closely with a client who had a lot of turbulence in her life. There were struggles in her relationships with family. She was unsatisfied at work because she felt she was being boxed into a certain role rather than allowed to grow. One day I woke up to find she had sent me six text messages during the night. She told me she was sinking under the overwhelming weight of other people's view of her. She needed to change something but she didn't know what or how. This was in the middle of the Covid crisis and it didn't feel like a good time for her to be making big decisions. It was so hard to evaluate all the uncertainty, she told me, and she was becoming very unhappy and anxious.

I've been working with this young woman for years and we know each other well. She takes her yoga practice very seriously and I could see, as I read the messages, that she was moving towards a point of clarity on her own. In the final message she said, 'I'm back to myself now. I've remembered that it's OK not to know. Thank you!'

There was no need to thank me – I did nothing at all. Nothing. But I was so pleased that she had found her own way to this point because it seemed to me exactly the most helpful place she could have ended up. She was embracing the education in life that circumstances were offering her and in doing so, she had returned to herself.

This return to self is deeply empowering and so liberating. When we embrace not knowing what's going on or what we should do, we open up to figuring it out from a place of deep authenticity. With the reduction in agitation that brings, our freedom for action increases.

There are three reasons to say 'I don't know'. First, because you really don't know, and that's OK. Second, when what you do know could really hurt someone if you say it. Thirdly, the 'I don't know' that keeps a situation on track and avoids going off at a tangent. Next time you're asked a question, might it be possible to create some space when you don't have an answer? Rather than look for a longer response, you could just say, 'I don't know.' In that way, you become a point of stability in the world, rather than adding to the chaos. In life, of course, you should always help where you can, but you can also experiment with 'I don't know' in different situations.

Clarity comes through action (2.26)

Have you ever had a friend who asks for your advice but never acts on it? Let's say you meet to discuss their difficulty with a new partner and spend hours talking over the problem, exploring interpretations and evaluating what to do. At the end of the evening your friend seems to have gained a lot of clarity. They've decided on a course of action and promise to get started the following morning. After all, as they admit, something has to change. But when you call them a couple of days later they haven't even spoken to their partner. They haven't done anything at all. They're stuck back in indecision or denial. If this cycle of planning for change only to fall back into inaction happens often enough, it's going to feel frustrating for both of you.

It's the same with your own life. You need a combination of reflection (through meditation) and action in order to decrease your unhappiness or struggle and bring about positive change. Meditation is the route for you to give yourself advice, just as you give it to your friends. It is a way to open up to your own insights. But those insights need to be tested in real life for effective change to occur.

This *sūtra* describes the concept of *viveka*, which is the power and courage of putting the clarity we have into action. When we follow a thought with action, we stress-test it and so gain more clarity for the next step. If we don't follow this process, as in the example of our friend who never puts advice into practice, then nothing will ever change and we will be stuck with a vague desire to sort out a relationship or move to the country or whatever it is we think we probably need to do but can't quite figure out. There is always work involved in bringing a plan to fruition. None of us can snap our fingers and conjure up what we want. That's not authentic change; it's just sleight of hand.

Build into your practice some periods for reflection through meditation so that you can open up to your own best advice. Then commit step by step, following through without rushing. So you act with clarity – *viveka*. (There are detailed suggestions for how to go about it in the next *sūtra*, which is the final one we'll be looking at in this section of the book.) Remember, you need to adopt both these complementary approaches to the gathering and accessing of wisdom in order for your life to change.

> *Meditation is inner clarity.* Viveka *is proof of our clarity to act in life. Without thinking, what's the best choice to make in a situation? What was your initial feeling about what to do? Can you trust that? What steps do you need to put in place to make it happen? Make sure that your actions in the right direction are achievable. Successes, however small, will build your confidence.*

A seven-step process for gaining clarity through action (2.27)

First, a quick reminder: the reason to do this work is the same reason for all yoga practice – to reduce your difficulties and increase your freedom to enjoy life. Now we've got that nailed down, let's look at how you can practise *viveka*. We're going to use the example of a couple who have two pre-school children and who tend to fight the moment they get home from work.

1. The first step towards solving any problem is always to ask yourself, 'What's the reality of the scenario I'm facing?' You're trying to get past what I call your personal propaganda, which is made up of your emotions and the story you're telling about the issue. You need to walk around it and assess it in a neutral way rather than falling for a projection – which could be your own but could also be somebody else's. This step is essentially a fact-finding mission, so you need to ask lots of questions. Using our example, you would need to ask what happens and when. Is there a row every day or only sometimes? What are the results? Does everybody end up angry or only one person? Then move from assessing the external facts to looking honestly at what you bring to the situation. Try to recognize what you really want, need and fear at every stage of the argument: in the build up, during and afterwards. Try to do this without judgement. This is about taking a look at what's really going on in order to gain maximum clarity. Without this understanding it's impossible to make changes.

2. After the fact-finding neutrality of the 'what', 'where' and 'when' questions, it's time to ask some 'why' questions. Ask yourself why this happens. What are

the triggers, for you and for your partner? Again, try to do this with as little blaming or judgement as possible. Perhaps one of you gets triggered by the other's habit of only texting to say they're going to be late at the time you were expecting them home. Perhaps one of you likes the kids rushing to greet them as they step through the door and the other needs five minutes of quiet space before they go and play with the children. Sometimes the trigger might simply be that one of you has had a particularly bad day and is taking it out on the other. The purpose of this stage of the work is to identify and take responsibility for the cause(s) of the fights, in order to try to avoid them in the future. Both partners need to do this. The aim is not to win an argument or cast blame. The aim is always to reduce future conflict.

3. OK, enough fact-finding, reflection and responsibility-taking. In order to move on you need action that takes you in a useful direction. You need an achievable and mutually agreed goal. That might be having dinner together at least three nights a week, so you can discuss life rather than fight over it. It might be as simple as going for a walk together.

4. Sounds great, but if it were as easy as goal-setting you'd already be doing it, right? True. So now we need to come up with the steps and tools that might make this happen. In this case, perhaps the returning partner agrees that they will always text as soon as they realize they're going to be late. Preferences over

noisy greetings on arrival or five minutes' calm will be respected.

5. The next stage is to put your agreed-upon steps and tools into practice. You need to try them out, calmly and in the spirit of hopeful curiosity.

6. Now, evaluate. You could do this over dinner. Do things feel easier? Are you having fewer arguments at 6 p.m.? If not, don't panic. Ask yourselves, 'How can we tweak this?' 'What else could we could try?' Accept that you might have to explore lots of different tools and even go back to step one and start again, in search of more clarity.

7. Step 7 is the resolution.

But if you do this work, steps 1 to 6, in good faith and as many times as necessary, then one day . . . You will walk through the front door after work, see your partner's shoulders slumped, feel your own mood fizzle and, rather than get irritated, you will know what to do to make things better for both of you, without resentment. You will have figured out, through trial and error, what interactions will help to boost you both. You will do them, and your partner's back will straighten. You'll smile at each other. Congratulations! You are now *viveka* champions, masters of clarity in action. (NB: I'm afraid you won't get to step 7 every time. It isn't the inevitable reward of running steps 1–6. But every time you do this work you'll get closer, and that will feel good. Closer is good enough.)

Exercise to develop clarity in action

Read the description above of the seven-step process of embedding *viveka* or clarity in action, with an example from your own life in mind. It could be an argument you've had recently, an encounter with somebody that upset you or a disappointing outcome at work, such as missing out on a promotion.

In the example above, some of the work involves discussing events with your partner. If you are focusing on an interaction with somebody else, it may be appropriate for you to discuss the seven-step process with them. If your focus is an interaction with an idea or event or object (missing the promotion, say) you might prefer to come up with your tools and strategies alone.

Take your time to run through the steps and map your experience onto each one in turn. I suggest you do this once to get events straight in your mind and then do it again, slowly, as you sit in meditation.

As you recall what happened for the second time, sit with each memory or idea and each feeling as it comes up. Don't rush from one to the next. Notice what surfaces from your mind. Don't accept your initial thoughts as being the final word. Dig a little deeper. Consider your motivation during these events. Think back to your actions and reactions. Look at them as honestly as you can. When emotions arise, notice without attaching a story to them.

Meditating on *viveka* in this way will involve drawing on everything we've discussed in the book so far. Think of it as a guided voyage of discovery into your mind. Anything and everything you find there is absolutely fine. There's no way to get this wrong. Just give it a go.

Thanks for sticking with me this far. You've come a really long way on your yoga journey. You're beginning to understand how this approach to your mind and to your interactions with other people can support you to live with less conflict and more freedom to be yourself. I hope you've been able to put in place a short daily practice of morning and evening yoga, using the breathing and meditation exercises from this chapter. And with the last section on clarity in action, you're starting to appreciate just how practical and far-reaching yoga can be.

I still get excited when somebody begins to really feel the relationship between the wisdom of the *Yoga Sūtra* and the possibility of transformation in their own life. It's such a beautiful symbiotic link. Rather than cause and effect ('Do yoga, get happy') it's a graceful spiral of feedback and interaction. You learn, you change, you learn more, you change again until you find that you are able to live with greater clarity than you ever imagined was possible. You are on your way to becoming a clear shining version of yourself, beaming your light into the world.

Let's keep going. In the next chapter I'll be showing you more practical tools to incorporate learning through yoga into your everyday life. And then we'll be spiralling upwards in search of more wisdom . . .

4. *Practical Yoga for Lifelong Change*

In this chapter we will be building on the foundations you've laid with your daily practice and exploring how to extend your learning as far as you wish to take it. We'll begin by recapping the tools in our yoga kit and practising an exercise related to each one. We'll also cover yoga's codes for positive living, in relation to yourself and other people, and look at them as frameworks for learning. There's a section on how yoga can support you when you encounter difficulties in your practice, as you inevitably will.

Since creating beneficial change takes a lot of faith – in ourselves and in what we're trying to do – we will also look at a particularly fascinating and challenging group of *sūtra* about what we believe in, which take us to the heart of yoga's most esoteric wisdom.

Finally, we'll loop back to explore meditation one last time before we finish our reading of the first two chapters of *Yoga Sūtra*. Since yoga is simply another name for meditation, it's fitting to end there. In reality, of course, there is no end to our journey towards yoga, so perhaps it's more accurate to say that it's a great place to pause or begin!

Group 11: Tools and techniques you can rely on

Keep breathwork as the basis of your practice (1.34)

Hopefully, you are now doing a breathing exercise every day, either in the morning or in the evening, or perhaps both. I hope that you are already seeing the benefits of bringing awareness to your breathing. There are so many reasons to practise *prāṇāyāma*, as we saw in the previous chapter. It reduces agitation and relieves pressure in the moment; it builds our confidence and self-reliance. And its benefits arrive quickly.

But the message of this *sūtra* is not that breathwork should be the basis of your practice, or that it's one of the most profound elements of self-care (though both those things are true). For me, the core message is about keeping on with what's working and what's essential, rather than flitting onto the latest new thing.

Yoga tells us that there's no single right way to do yoga, and that we must each find our own path. But this *sūtra* also tells us that there is value in deepening our commitment to what works for us once we've found it. Many times it's powerful to combine different elements, techniques and concepts of yoga, or indeed to practise yoga alongside other healing approaches. But not always. Sometimes we need to deepen our practice rather than broaden it. And we need to be patient enough to explore aspects of yoga fully before we move on. We would do well to keep our focus on breathing, even as we add in posture work or more meditations or mantras or further study. In this way we keep the faith with our own practice, and that's one of the most important and powerful approaches of all.

Have you noticed any changes in your emotional state since you've been doing breathwork? They might be very much in the moment or more pervasive. Seek out what's changed for you and, with that clear focus in your mind, commit to working with your breath on an ongoing basis.

Exercise to reduce stress and anxiety

This exercise introduces an element of simple physical practice to your breathing work and focuses on the incredible benefits of exhalation. It is one of the most effective tools I know for maintaining calm, even as life becomes stressful or complex. I rely on it every day and I can't imagine being without it. Once you've got the habit, I suspect you'll feel the same.

1. Take some free breaths and check in with yourself to see how you're feeling. Then take some long regular breaths to prepare. Let your breathing slow as you begin to focus on it.

2. Now take hold of your nose with your thumb and forefinger, just below the bridge and close to the bone but where it's still squidgy enough to pinch the

nostrils closed. Pinch once to check your fingers are in the right place, but then unpinch and just rest your fingers there. Relax your shoulders and drop your chin a little. Try not to tense your neck or arm.

3. Take a long slow breath in through both nostrils. Then pinch your right nostril shut using as little force as possible and exhale consistently and slowly through your left nostril.
4. Release the nostril at the end of your out-breath and take another slow in-breath through both nostrils. This time you're going to close the left nostril and exhale gently through the right one.
5. Do this six times on the right and six times on the left in total, alternating. If you need to take a few free breaths in between, please do. The aim is to breathe in a rhythm that is sustainable for you without straining or holding your breath. Don't force anything.
6. Finish with a few more free breaths, keeping them long, slow and steady, just as you did at the beginning of the exercise. Notice your state of mind now. Has it changed? This checking-out process will help you to mitigate any mistakes such as rushing or holding your breath.
7. With practice, you can build up to eight, ten, twelve or more repetitions, but do this over a period of weeks rather than days.

Get used to regular sanity checking (1.35)

An improved objective perception of reality is fundamental to yoga, but complete objectivity is not a realistic aim, as you know. Better simply to commit to regular work to clear away the biases and outdated beliefs, assumptions and errors of judgement that cloud our reading of a situation.

As we've seen already, the way to do this is to disengage gently from our reactions to whatever it is we're seeing, hearing, touching, etc. Our brain relies on our sense organs to gather up information about the outside world. It then turns those signals into meanings, thoughts, ideas and emotions. Most of us, especially at the beginning of our yoga practice, are slaves to our senses. It's a really good habit to practise sanity checking our reactions whenever we feel ourselves getting unstable or uncomfortable. The way to do this is simply to pause and ask a question. It might be as simple as, 'What's really going on here?' or, 'What do I know for sure?' It could be, 'Where's my anxiety coming up from?' or, 'Why do I want this?' The question is not as important as the habit of asking. Every time you stop to question your immediate responses to an object that your sense organs are telling you about, you are training your mind and moving closer to yoga.

The next time a voice pipes up in your head, whether it's critical or self-pitying or self-satisfied, can you ignore the content and just register it as an opportunity to practise? What are the facts? How to stick to the reality? Can you qualify what's memory and what's imagination? What is it you don't know?

Exercise to get better at pausing before you react

This practice is divided into two parts. Firstly, you're going to recall a situation or object that got you into a difficult or uncomfortable state of mind recently. It could be a gossipy conversation or a snide comment you or someone else made. It could be your decision to drink yet another large glass of wine.

Once you've picked your sticky situation, recall how you felt. Try to remember your state of mind and emotions before, during and afterwards. Were you bored, angry, tired, resentful? Why? Where had those thoughts and feelings come from? Was your inner critic on full rant mode that day? Had you woken up feeling exhausted by a night of bad dreams? Investigate. Return in your memory to the glass of wine or the comment you regret, and pause. Imagine yourself in that split second beforehand and just rest there. Listen to any comments in your mind, any feelings that come up. You're noticing them, nothing else.

The second part of the exercise is to repeat this with an imagined sticky situation that hasn't happened yet but could. It could be very similar to the first incident, with the same trigger. Imagine yourself in that split second before the drink or the sarcastic comment. Pause. Rest there, holding this moment in your mind's eye.

The aim is to practise using our powers of both memory and imagination so that it gradually becomes easier to pause in the moment in real time. Eventually, you will be able to pause and sanity check your actions and reactions with ease. In the meantime, don't worry if this is a struggle.

It might help to regard every emotion that comes up, even the uncomfortable ones, as your trigger to learn. These moments are not obstacles but opportunities. The task is not to banish the inner critic completely (fat chance!) but to notice its presence without paying attention to its words.

Choose to focus on the lighter side (1.36)

Our reaction to events determines their impact on us even more than the event itself. Say you get down to the final two at interview and then miss out on the job. You're certainly going to be disappointed. You might feel angry or fret over the things you should have done differently. If you choose to interpret it as evidence that you're not good enough to succeed at anything, you are heading for self-recrimination and hostility, bitterness and low mood. If, on the other hand, you can congratulate yourself for having got so close, you lessen your distress and set yourself up for better luck next time. It might take a day or three to get to that accepting place, but once the first disappointment has passed, what happens next is a question of which story you decide to tell yourself. It is a choice.

I'm not saying that all you need to do is look on the bright side. That's just denial of the reality of feelings and doesn't help anyone. One of the first principles in yoga is that your experience is meaningful and your feelings are valid. So, take your time to feel the necessary feelings of sadness or anger, but detach as gently as you can, as soon as you can, and get on with the business of integrating what's helpful and turning away from what isn't. In my experience, there are very few situations in life that cannot be made worse by choosing to see them as a disaster that you either didn't deserve or brought on yourself.

Sometimes, of course, bad things do happen to us. We will all lose people we love, for example. But even the most tragic or traumatic event can be made more or less painful by how we process our grief and how we frame what happened. The greater the pain, the more work will be required to release grief and make meanings that support us.

The first step in any situation is to recognize that when we have been hurt or disappointed there is no shortcut to feeling better. We cannot bypass the reality of our situation, which includes our painful feelings. We must release them with tears, or a chat with a friend, or whatever method brings us relief.

The second step is to distinguish between the reality that requires our attention and whatever we are bringing in terms of interpretation. Our memories are always keen to bring in comparisons. Our imaginations chip in with ideas about how this will play out in the future. These contributions might be helpful or unhelpful, but, either way, they are elements that we are responsible for bringing. They are different from and additional to the reality. (There is an exercise at the end of this section to help you investigate this process.) Once we've teased apart what's real, what's unknown and what's simply unknowable, we can see that the object we have to contend with has become smaller. It's still there – you still didn't get that job – but without our catastrophic story, its enormity has shrunk to a much more manageable size.

This allows your mind to calm down. Once in this calmer state, you're ready for the final step, which is to arrive at the lightest possible way to interpret events. This is not about denial of reality; it's more about choosing not to catastrophize. Turning your attention towards the light rather than the dark.

It's about taking charge of your feelings and your interpretations and doing more of what will benefit rather damage you. As the clouds break on a stormy afternoon and the rain soaks your clothes you might be treated to a rainbow sparkling bright against the grey clouds. It's true that you're wet and starting to get cold. It's also true that the sky is beautiful, and your flat is only ten minutes away. Which will you choose to focus on as you hurry home? The light or the dark?

Do you believe that pain and grief are unacceptable or unbearable? Or do you believe that they're normal, inevitable, parts of life? Can you embrace that both light and dark are part of you, and that that's OK?

Exercise for making healthier interpretations

Our previous exercise looked at cultivating that tiny, crucial pause that allows you the distance you need to respond rather than react to situations. We're building on that work here by looking at ways you can strengthen your ability to differentiate between the facts of a situation – let's say, you've failed an exam – and the additional elements that might be increasing your unhappiness as you begin to consider what this outcome might mean for you.

This *sūtra* (1.36) tells us that there are three additional elements at play. We have our memories and imaginations, which are doing their jobs by pushing various interpretations at us. For example, you might recall a story your father once told you about a friend who didn't gain his qualifications to become a lawyer and whose life took a different (less successful) turn from the one he'd hoped for. Such stories are highly unlikely to make us feel better about our situation, and yet they are bound to crop up because memory is just doing what it's designed to do. Imagination, meanwhile, might pitch in with another unhelpful suggestion: that your exam failure has just doomed you to miss out on the crucial promotion and suffer years of stagnation at work, boredom, frustration, the end of your relationship, a drink problem and eventually total and abject failure in every aspect of life. (Thanks, imagination.)

The third element is not so much what we're bringing as what we're missing. Not-knowing is the elephant in the room. To what extent could we see our situation clearly? What were we unable to see? When you failed that exam, did you really know enough to interpret the implications? Almost certainly not. So perhaps you could have stepped away from interpretation and returned to the bare reality. You didn't pass. What next? Not-knowing could be a friend here, if we let it.

Prepare yourself for the next time a difficult situation occurs in your life by looking back to something that worried you at the time but which turned out to be a non-event.

Can you see, with hindsight, the difference between the reality and the interpretive work of your memory and imagination? Can you see the element of not-knowing and see how you rushed to fill it with interpretation rather than treat it as your opportunity to do something different? Can you recall what it felt like to be in the middle of the difficult situation? What were your feelings and thoughts? Can you recall any of the language you used to describe what was going on, to yourself or others?

Now, remember when your view shifted and you were able to see the event as non-threatening. What changed? How did you feel? Did a friend offer a different interpretation, perhaps? Did time pass? Did you face the event and get through it without disaster? Try to meditate on how you were interpreting in the moment when you realized that whatever you had worried about had passed, without catastrophe. Conjure up those feelings of relief.

The more often you can visualize yourself in that state of clear-sighted calm, the better. You are reminding yourself that your mind can be peaceful. From this peace, it can reach for the lightest interpretation possible. This will make it easier to frame an uncertain or challenging situation neutrally, or lightly, without denying those elements of it that cause you pain.

Get to know your inner diva (1.37)

You're probably familiar with the idea of the 'inner critic', that nasty internal voice that loves to point out your flaws and failings. Needless to say, yoga has no time for inner critics. I used to know mine very well, but I don't hear from it much these days and, when it does turn up, I can dismiss it pretty quickly. I know it's just remnants of old fear, desires, anger and sadness. I would encourage you to meditate on recognizing your own version of that voice and realizing that it has no reality or power whatsoever, except that which you give it.

I would also encourage you to listen out for another internal voice: the one that this *sūtra* addresses. As well as the inner critic, many of us have an inner narcissist, or an inner diva. This is the voice of our desires, our sense of entitlement, our ego. It says things like, 'I deserve . . .' 'I demand that you . . .' 'I want, I need . . .' It is not the calm and centred yoga mind that knows itself intimately and honestly and can insist on its right to be respected without ever raising its voice. It's a shrill and needy call that embodies our most self-centred mindset.

In this *sūtra* we're encouraged to deal with that desiring, grasping, clinging mind. It asks us to get better at answering the questions, 'Why am I holding on to this so hard?' 'How much pushing is too much for this outcome that I'm so attached to?' 'What is motivating my actions?' (Usually the answer is 'I want attention / to be seen / heard / held.') There's definitely something of the toddler to our inner diva!

How can you stop using drama to distract yourself from what you really need? One simple question to begin this dialling down is to ask yourself whether you are tired or hungry. Drama increases when we don't listen to our bodies' signals. What is it that you are you holding on to? And why?

Exercise for recognizing your inner diva

Set an intention today to listen out for the words and tones your inner diva prefers. Whenever you hear yourself saying or thinking things like, 'I deserve to have . . .' or, 'He should give me . . .' or, 'That's not fair!' it's a clue that your inner diva has taken over. Its shrill, foot-stamping tone is a sign that you're deep in a desiring mindset.

Don't worry if you don't notice what's going on until after an inner tantrum. This exercise isn't easy, and hindsight is the most helpful tool we have when we're doing this kind of work. You will get better at noticing and gently detaching from your diva's demands, but it takes practice to attune your ear to its language.

Once you've built some skill at noticing what your diva's up to, ask yourself how often you externalize these feelings and act them out with other people. Are there certain people who seem to unleash it? Are there specific situations in which it's almost guaranteed to show up? Try not to blame yourself or others; just notice. This is the start of powerful change.

Let your dreaming mind teach you intuition (1.38)

How to get a good night's sleep? Judging by the number of people I talk to who ask me this question, it seems there's an epidemic of sleep disorders out there. The damaging effects of insomnia or broken nights on our physical, mental and emotional wellbeing are well known, and yet many of us struggle to establish habits that make it easier for us to get the rest we need.

Yoga is one of the most effective things you can do to

improve your sleep. If you're waking a lot during the night or you find your mind racing the moment your head touches the pillow, then a late-night practice, just before bed, should be a first port of call. I find it especially effective to work with that busy mind rather than fight it. On nights when I'm struggling to drift off, I thank my mind for doing its job: planning, processing and generally trying to be useful and keep me safe. Its timing might be off but its intentions are sound. Once I've acknowledged its work I find it easier to turn my focus elsewhere and meditate on something restful.

Beyond these practical ways that yoga can support sleep, there is an insight contained in this *sūtra* that is deeply powerful, though a little esoteric. According to yoga, your dreaming mind is distinct from your sleeping mind, and, just as with your meditating mind, you can learn from it. When we dream, our minds are free to roam in a realm that is unbound by the usual constraints of physical reality. The effects of imagination and memory upon our brains' functioning are different. The dreaming mind is free to reassess and reorder events, to act out a scenario that would be impossible in the waking world and for the everyday mindset.

Dreams are a vehicle for intuition. When we recall something from a dream we are receiving a message from an area of the mind that is usually inaccessible when we are awake. I'm not suggesting that we could or should decode our dreams for their specific secret meanings, but I do think we can learn to open up to the insights they offer us. For example, if you have a dream that upsets you about someone or something that you have told yourself you're not bothered about, that might be a sign to pay some more attention. Focus on the event or person in your next mediation and see what comes up. If you allow your dreams to support you in this way, they can become great allies.

Can you contemplate taking your dreams seriously? You don't need to try to decode them, just pay attention to them. Is there coincidence in life? Does everything have a reason? What lessons can you get from your dreams? What can you learn from your sleep process?

Exercise to disengage from sleeplessness

Rather than treating good sleep as yet another task and sleeplessness as the enemy, can you practise thinking of both sleep and sleeplessness as opportunities to rest and to learn? This is not easy for anyone who has regularly suffered the distress of not being able to get to or stay asleep, and it's essential to support your mind to disengage from its negative associations.

Begin this visualization exercise when you're feeling well rested and are not stressed about sleep. Pick the moment in your day when you feel most alert.

Settle yourself comfortably, either lying down or sitting either cross-legged on the floor or in a chair with both your feet resting on the floor and your hands gently on your knees or in your lap. Close your eyes and take some long, smooth breaths. Feel your mind settling.

When you're ready, visualize the next moment of wakefulness that you're going to experience. Imagine yourself waking up in the middle of the night. Acknowledge how you typically react to this, perhaps with irritation or even panic, by lying in the dark ruminating or by turning the light on to read or getting up. Acknowledge what happens and look not to get involved with your usual story about it. So no rehearsing any worries about how you will cope the following day, for example. Instead, imagine doing something different. If you never get up, imagine getting out of bed and moving to another room to do a short breathing practice before returning to bed. See yourself resting your mind in breath then returning to bed and falling asleep. Alternatively, try visualizing yourself cutting your normal narrative before you begin your involvement with it. Thank your mind for what it's doing, ask it to continue its good work while you go back to sleep.

In this way you are rehearsing strategies for the next time you need them and preparing your mind not to panic but to see that moment of wakefulness as just another interlude in your life. You are supporting yourself to nip sleeplessness in the bud and move through it as peacefully as possible.

Treat meditation seriously and it will reward you (1.39)

This is an interesting *sūtra*. Its literal meaning is (approximately), 'Meditate on something that you find agreeable.' But agreeable in this context doesn't translate to 'easy'. The *Yoga Sūtra* is not urging us to use meditation as a way to chill out or relax. It would be more accurate to interpret this line as a reminder that meditation can be as rewarding and as life-changing as you make it. When we meditate upon something nutritious for our minds, we begin to develop a two-way relationship between our selves and the object. This is an active process that we instigate and participate in fully. One classic example would be meditating on a proverb or mantra, exploring its richness and significance.

The aim of this kind of meditation is not so much to calm the mind (though obviously there's nothing wrong with that) but to go further. For example, it can support you in not getting too involved with your emotions. You might decide to review a moment of irritation during a meditation session. Hold it in the back of your mind while you focus your attention on a mantra. This can strengthen your capacity to be aware of your emotions without being wrapped up in them. This sort of meditation practice encourages us to seek out our own internal supports, build our resilience and reduce our dependency on external crutches.

For me, this *sūtra* expresses the difference in value between using a guided meditation on an app for ten minutes and building up the confidence and strength of mind to practise solo meditation for half an hour. To be clear, I'm not saying there's anything wrong with guided meditation or meditation apps, especially when we're new to yoga, but what this *sūtra* reminds me is that meditation practice can always take us a little further. There are no limits on your own mind if you commit to exploring it fully.

Can you meditate on something that attracts you or that you love to help you feel more peaceful? If you already meditate, can you open up to re-examining meditation's place in your life? There is no one right way to meditate. What's yours?

Exercise to strengthen your capacity to meditate

This simple tool uses your voice to produce an object for meditation while you do some breathwork. So we're combining two elements here – the breathing and the voice – but in a very simple way. Use the letter A as your object, and just say Aaaaaaaaaa softly and with equal consistency every time you breathe out. You can say it out loud if you feel comfortable doing so, or in your head.

Find yourself a comfortable place to sit and take some long, slow preparatory breaths. When you feel your mind settling enough to begin, introduce the voicework. Repeat ten times, with ten accompanying breaths. Observe how your mind behaves as you repeat the sound. When you get to the end of this set of ten, stop and sit in silence, focusing on your breath, and see what comes up. Then do another set of ten.

You may feel a bit silly. Don't worry if you do, just notice and keep on breathing and saying this simple sound.

Do this exercise every day for a week and observe any changes in your mind. If you would like to introduce a movement as well at the end of the week, feel free. Any simple movement that feels easy to you is fine, with the sound on the exhale of the movement.

Try to be aware of the distance and difference between your breathing, movement and voicework. Do you tend to focus on one more than the others? Do you find one element much more difficult than the others? This is fine. Just keep observing. After a certain amount of practice you may notice that, although each element remains present, none is dominating your reactions. (Or you may not!)

Practise the art of getting unstuck (1.40)

There will always be moments when you get hung up on something. None of us is completely immune to the objects that hook us in and make us crazy, however much yoga we practise. Whether it's salt-and-vinegar crisps, your mother's barbed comments about your parenting or an old and painful memory, there's likely to be something that can still make you react in a hurry and get lost in emotion.

This *sūtra* tells us that what we need in these moments is the ability to stay dynamic. To shift our perspective from close-up observation and detail to gentle disengagement and greater perspective (or the other way round), in a movement as fluid and unforced as when we breathe. When we are able to move smoothly between these two positions in relation to any object, however hooky, we have mastered the art of getting unstuck.

During one particular training session in India when I was studying to be a yoga therapist, I was invited by TKV to participate in a consultation with a patient. He would conduct the session alongside another trainee, much more experienced than me, who was also a doctor of conventional medicine. At the end of the session, I would be asked for my diagnostic opinion and suggestions for treatment. I felt honoured to be invited but also intimidated, desperate to learn and to show how much I knew.

When the day came, I was terribly nervous. The patient arrived and I stood at the back of the room, clutching a notebook and pencil, as TKV began to speak with him. I hadn't been told anything about the man's condition or history so I scanned his body, his posture and demeanour as he and TKV chatted for a minute about this and that. I barely listened as I scribbled notes and waited for the consultation to really begin.

So imagine my shock when TKV said goodbye to the patient and left. We hadn't even started! I began to sweat.

Next up was the doctor, who seemed much more relaxed than I was. He asked a great many questions. I felt my anxiety rising as I struggled to process what I was hearing and observing. My heart was sinking as I felt this opportunity going to waste. Eventually, the doctor turned to me and asked me for my thoughts. 'What would you suggest for this patient, Colin?' My mind went blank. 'I'm not sure,' I said. 'Could I let you know tomorrow?'

As soon as I'd spoken, I felt ridiculous. The patient was right here, in front of me. He needed direction now – not tomorrow.

The doctor smiled kindly and turned back to the patient to make suggestions. I listened in, but my heart was sinking. What would everyone think of me?

When we spoke afterwards, TKV was as unruffled and reassuring as always. He helped me to see that the primary learning for me in this situation was not how to diagnose and treat a patient but how to detach from my own agenda enough to be fully present. To hone in on detail and then pause, track out again and think. Unhook from any *kleśa* that were rushing in to take up space in my thinking mind, whether that be my ego's desire to impress, or my fear of getting things wrong. Once detached, I could return to the level of detail, take another look, have another think and so on.

This dynamic movement between perspectives allows for better understanding, but it is a skill that requires practice. TKV had taken one glance at our patient and was able to see almost immediately what was going on and what would help. The doctor took his time to listen to and observe the person in front of him. I, on the other hand, had been caught on the hook of my desire to please. I got lost in my needs at the expense of my own learning and the patient's wellbeing. I had frozen completely.

If I had stayed stuck, wriggling on the hook of my ego's bruising, I would have learned nothing at all. Luckily, I had learned just enough to detach myself and keep the incident in perspective. It's a lesson I still have to practise but have never forgotten.

Today, set an intention to look out for any moments in which you think a variation on either, 'I give up' or, 'I have to double down and get this sorted.' This sort of language reveals that we are moving either away from or towards an object in an uncontrolled and emotional manner. This is a sign that we're on the brink of missing an opportunity to practise a more fluid shift in perspective. How can you get an overall view of the situation as well as being able to go into the detail?

Exercise to increase your comfort with shifting perspectives

You can do this exercise to prepare yourself for the next time you need to either zoom in and look clearly at the detail of a situation, or step back and consider the bigger picture. The ability to shift smoothly and easily between close-up and big picture is one of the most fundamental skills we must all work on if we want our minds to evolve. It's very common to parachute out of difficult situations or, conversely, to get bogged down in their minutiae and end up obsessing over the 'he said . . .' and 'she said . . .'. We can all learn to be more in control of where we're standing in relation to events, and in this way alter our perspective in helpful rather than harmful directions.

You're going to recall a time recently when you justified yourself to somebody during the course of a disagreement. Perhaps you said something like, 'I only did it because I thought you would like it.' The form of the words and the context don't matter. What you're looking for is the kind of language that gives you the clue that you were getting bogged down in petty detail rather than asking bigger questions that would pull you out to greater clarity. In the context of our hypothetical disagreement, for example, it might have been better to pause, step back and consider the bigger picture. Is the relationship with this person no longer healthy? Rather than justify yourself, would you be better off reframing the relationship or even shifting out of it altogether? Or on the other hand, if the relationship *is* important and healthy, perhaps a bigger-picture perspective on the incident or behaviour you were trying to justify shows you that you should simply have apologized and moved on.

Next, look for an incident in your recent life when you can see that you were a bit too disengaged rather than over-engaged. How can you tell? Can you identify the moment when you could have changed the outcome by coming closer and tackling a salient detail?

The more you can review your interactions in this way and spot which direction you were travelling in and what results you got, the more skilled you will be at noticing in real time and either stepping back or stepping in as required.

Group 12: How to get success and clarity in your relationships

This section of the *Yoga Sūtra* is unusually direct in its instructions on how to practise and how to refine our behaviour more generally. The first *sūtra* lists the eight core components of the yoga process. The next five *sūtra* lay out in detail the mechanics of behavioural attitudes that make up the first two components: *yama* (outward-facing interactions with our environment, other people, etc.) and *niyama* (inward-facing interactions between aspects of our own selves).

It can be tempting to treat all this as a set of rules for how yoga wants you to live your life, or a checklist of goals to tick off on your yoga journey. Tempting, but not that helpful. Unlike the Ten Commandments of Judaism and Christianity, these *sūtra* are not 'given by God'. Yoga does not judge as sinful people who don't follow them, because yoga doesn't talk about morality. So this is not about being a 'good' or 'bad' person. It's through this process that we can refine practising our internal and external relationships to achieve more success in daily life.

I think of these *sūtra* as pointers towards a life that features less ego and more genuine personality, less talking and more listening. Not because living in this way makes you more worthy but because it is likely to reduce both your own personal issues and the amount of suffering in the world. To me, these *sūtra* read like guidelines for living a more comfortable and stable life that makes a positive contribution to the common good. There's a strong imperative in the way they're set out, mind you. They might not be rules, they're definitely not commandments, but perhaps they form a code of ethical conduct (voluntary, of course) that promises to give a deep and continuous clarity and allow you to shine. Could be worthwhile?

Eight components of yoga – use with caution (2.29)

Here comes a list. It's not in order of priorities, and it's not a route map to enlightenment, but it does start from foundational practices and progress through to the most advanced and esoteric. On that note, this *sūtra* makes clear that the foundations of yoga are all about our relationships, with self and other. But do remember that our learning is not linear and all of us will need to grow outwards and inwards. It might help to think of this list as a framework for how to learn about the world and yourself.

1. *Yama* – refining of our outward-looking attitudes, actions and reactions.
2. *Niyama* – refining of our inward-looking attitudes, actions and reactions.
3. *Āsana* – the practice of physical postures.
4. *Prāṇāyāma* – the practice of breathing exercises.
5. *Pratyāharā* – ability to be the director of our senses.
6. *Dhāraṇā* – the capacity to direct and focus our minds.

7. *Dhyāna* – the ability to understand an object through meditation.
8. *Samādhi* – integration with the object we're trying to understand.

Yama: *attitudes that help with relationships out in the world* (2.30)

1. Respect all living things. Understand the principle of non-violence, which requires us to consider whether our behaviours cause distress to other creatures. Learning to apply it to everything you do, think and say.
2. Tell the truth, in your actions as well as your words. Work to understand that truth is not absolute; it is something you co-create with other people and with reality. How to do this without hurting others?
3. Finesse your attitudes to giving, taking and receiving. What do you consider as stealing or coveting what is not yours in your relationships? (It may well not be a material physical theft.)
4. Be measured, appropriate and boundaried in all your actions and relationships. Observe the energy you bring to situations. Notice whether you bring drama, apathy, a need to control, take over or avoid, or any other power dynamic.
5. Understand what you're grasping on to and striving for.

The five simple ideas in this *sūtra* remind us just how much we can learn by observing how we act around other people and also how they react to us. By being honest about your relationships and interactions with others. If you often get into arguments or do a lot for other people but resent it afterwards, those might be signs that your best starting point for exploration is *yama*.

Reflect on these five ideas in your daily life. What do they mean to you? How important are they to you? Can you start to see how all these attitudes and behaviours are interlinked in your own life?

How to have more success in your relationships (2.31)

There is a nugget of practical wisdom in this *sūtra* that helps us to understand and apply the previous one. It says that none of us should get too attached to our rules to live by because the volatility of nature means that everything is always changing. Add other people into the mix and things get even more unpredictable. Context is crucial to every single interaction we have with another person and with the world. What works in one situation will not necessarily work in another. The strategies that enable your friend to have a harmonious relationship with her mother, for example, might not work for you with yours. That may sound obvious, but it's amazing how often we forget it.

This *sūtra* reminds us to set a clear intention to be open-minded in all our interactions and attitudes, to respond rather than react, and be curious and patient. To work from the place we're in, right here and now. We all need to figure out our particular role and circumstances, as well as the other person's. Every single element in life is a variable that will affect our outcomes, so we will find life easier if we practise adaptability.

There's no magic formula for success, which makes life both more challenging and more exciting.

Can you adapt and change based on context? Can you remain open to the idea that you have something to learn in every situation? You have a new opportunity in every single moment and with every single interaction. What are you going to do with it?

Niyama: *attitudes that will help your relationship with yourself* (2.32)

1. How can you look after, maintain and evolve your body, mind and surroundings so that you get the best out of yourself? How can you reduce *kleśa* and keep yourself sane?
2. Be content with what you have and comfortable with what you lack. Embrace 'good enough' rather than aiming for non-existent perfection. When you do this you energize yourself to make sustainable progress.
3. Embrace discipline in your physical self-care. Sleep and eat well, do good work, take exercise and make time for relaxation.
4. Cultivate the habit of evaluating in order to improve. Check your progress in all areas. Be honest when you reflect on your actions.

5. Sometimes the best thing we can do is lighten up. Be kind to ourselves. Laugh a little. Surrender to acceptance. Remember, every moment is an opportunity to try a new approach, so how serious is any one moment, really?

Is it a challenge for you to care for yourself? Do you struggle to let go of mistakes, laugh at your foibles or move on from a bad day? These are all signs that your best starting point might be with *niyama*.

> *How honest are you being about how you treat yourself? If you resist the ideas of your* niyama, *ask yourself why.*

How to be considerate towards yourself and others (2.33)

In the same way that intention is important when we are using *yama* to learn through our interactions with the outside world, it is also important when we're using *niyama*. It's helpful if we can avoid treating *niyama* as a recipe for self-improvement – not least because there's nothing wrong with whoever you are right now – but instead use it as a framework for open-minded growth. In the same way that *yama* is a framework for learning through compassionate interactions with others, *niyama* is a framework for learning through compassionate and considerate interactions with yourself. The key to unlocking both of these approaches is the ability to cultivate perspectives that are different from those you currently hold.

Please don't worry if you're not yet practising these attitudes towards yourself or others. They can feel very challenging for some of us (and, if that's the case, all the more reason to start with them). If you can cultivate them you will see yourself more clearly. It will be easier to live as a comfortable and stable expression of who you really are.

Do you accept mediocrity or do you look to improve yourself anytime you can? Can you find the courage to be ready to healthily question yourself?

Yama *and* niyama *always operate in tandem* (2.34)

In the real world, our internal and external attitudes are constantly interacting. How we relate to ourselves establishes who we are. We then project that sense of self when we interact with other people and when they react to us. And, of course, everybody else is doing exactly the same thing at the same time.

If we can incorporate *yama* and *niyama* into as many of our everyday interactions as possible, we are likely to have a smoother time of it. Practical aspects of our existence, like decision-making, as well as emotional aspects, such as our relationships with family and friends, become easier. Over time we will have fewer messes to clear up or apologies to make. We will feel less resentful and more appreciated because we will have learned to consider our selves and others in a clear-sighted way, anticipate problems and avoid them.

A friend of mine was telling me recently what a struggle it is to react positively to her father. He constantly gripes about the way she's bringing up her children and can be very aggressive in his criticism. It's hard not to meet his aggression with her own anger. We explored what happens for her during these interactions. She recognized that she is holding on very tightly to the way she wants to be perceived, as a daughter and as a mother. She is also very attached to her idea of how a father and his grown-up daughter *should* be with one another. As a consequence, she goes into these encounters with a desired outcome that is not realistic. And while her attention is focused on this dynamic, she's not able to see the daily successes she has in her role as a mother, which is ultimately now a higher priority for her. Could she imagine a different outcome? One that embraced a meeting with the father she actually has, as the person she is? We agreed that she would set an intention to remember all these points as she arrived for her next visit to her dad.

We also talked about what it might mean to tell the truth that doesn't hurt in this context, as well as to behave in a measured and appropriate way – three of the codes of *yama*. My friend decided that telling the truth meant setting and communicating clear boundaries about the language and treatment she was prepared to accept from her father. Appropriate behaviour meant aiming to meet him with love but leaving his house if she could not (because he was overstepping her boundaries).

At the end of our chat she said something that I found very interesting. 'I want to learn how to handle this difficult situation,' she said. 'My dad's a grumpy old man but he won't be around for ever. I want to use this time to practise relating to him in ways that feel honest and appropriate. All I can do is try – and hope that he meets my efforts with his own.'

I agreed with her. I also reminded her that it might well be exhausting, so it would be a good idea to factor in some extra support and comfort for days when she was visiting her father. In that way she would be showing consideration towards herself as well as her grumpy old man.

To cultivate a different perspective, step through these questions: 1. What's the origin of the issue? Is it you? Someone acting on your behalf? Someone with no involvement to you? 2. What's your true motivation in this situation? Is there desire/greed? Are you angry? Is there delusion? 3. What's going to be the intensity of the outcome for you? A little pain? Quite a lot of grief? Huge suffering? 4. How do you choose a priority that brings more clarity, more knowledge and better relationships?

Group 13: Does your outward self match your inner one?

The idea of yoga being based on 'good' balance comes up a lot in people's understanding, but I think the concept of balance gets overplayed. If everything in life and our minds was really in a perfect state of balance there would be nothing but stasis. Literally, nothing going on.

There's one area of yoga where the balance image does come in useful, though, and that's when we're reflecting on how much coherence there is between our relationship with things 'out there' and our relationship with things 'in here', inside our own minds. The more consistency between the two, the more likely we are to be living in a comfortable and stable way that reflects who we are, both in the privacy of our own minds and out in the world.

As ever, this is not about success or failure. Many of us lack self-confidence, for example, so we project confidence that we don't feel. That doesn't make us a fake or a bad person, but it might not increase our stock of true confidence, either. Rather than projecting confidence we don't really feel, perhaps we could re-examine our feelings of under-confidence. Once we've noticed a mismatch in any area, it's important to first look inside rather than outside, and recalibrate our interactions with our critical thoughts or painful memories as gently as we can.

This section of the *Yoga Sūtra* works through each of the attitudes listed under *yama* and *niyama* and shows us how to spot signs of progress in cultivating each one. Each *sūtra* is balanced around a point of interaction between *yama* and *niyama*. Use the following lines to reflect on your yoga practice and its impact. They show us how to harness the insights we gain through our relationships to grow more fully into the essence of who we really are, and vice versa.

1. The more peaceful you are, the more peace you can transmit to others and the less likely you are to fall into the trap of mirroring negative states of mind (2.35).

How can you accept where someone else is at? How can you use a peaceful mindset to influence others? How can you use a positive attitude to disable something?

2. Beautiful honesty makes for healthy relationships. When you tell your truth with sensitivity, you make deeper connections (2.36).

Are you able to be honest in your relationships? That's honest as in able to express a multidimensional truth? How can you tell the truth that doesn't hurt? As well as the truth that's relative to them?

3. When you're neither greedy nor needy, generosity flows towards you (2.37).

Do you trust that there is enough and that life will flow towards you? How do you give just enough to others in each context and situation?

4. Strength is obtained through moderation, so be measured and consistent in your actions and relationships. If you are erratic or excessive or unengaged, it will make you weak (2.38).

How do you manage your energy on a daily basis? How to take the middle path of not too much and not too little? What can you learn about your own boundaries by watching other people set theirs, or not?

5. Clinging on to things takes time and energy away from the practice of asking whether they serve you (2.39).

What is it that you're really holding on to? What do you really want? If you ask enough times, patiently following the trail, you will find the origins of any issue.

6. As you refine your body and mind, you acquire the wisdom that shows you the difference between the external (which inevitably deteriorates) and that which is deep inside (and beyond decay) (2.40).

Can you turn the label you attach to your body (too fat, too thin), or to your mind (too boring, too fiery) into an opportunity for refinement? Can you drop the label?

7. Strive to distinguish between what you want and what you need; this wisdom leads away from suffering and towards contentment (2.41).

This is yoga in action. How can you interact with others efficiently and clearly with good feeling and focus? How can you deal with any situation always keeping a clear mind?

8. Contentment is a starting point on the journey to happiness but we need to refine our minds even to get there. We do this by cultivating the ability to expand or contract our energy and focus to meet life's demands as they arise: rules are less useful than flexibility (2.42).

Contentment is only the beginning and happiness is a by-product – they are not goals. How can you keep questioning and evolving when the going is good and you feel content?

9. Without discipline over the senses it's impossible to keep working towards greater understanding. Support

your practice and your health by working to be in charge of your impulses each and every day (2.43).

What is it that you reach for most habitually? How can you gently reduce your time on Instagram or the number of drinks you consume?

10. Self-inquiry shows us that we each have a light side and a dark one; it enables us to move towards the better version of our selves. It also shows us that there is something greater than us with which we can connect. Both strands of this inquiry will move us in a good direction (2.44).

Can you be open to understanding that there are different parts of yourself, without criticizing them? How can you create links and relationships with others that change distrust? How do you improve yourself so that your evolution is the proof of your success?

And the result and reward of incorporating all these attitudes is . . . true ability *(2.45)*.

Only through cultivating great respect for our selves, others and *Īśvara* (pronounced Eesh-vah-ra, 'the one who carries power', which we will cover in Group 15) can we integrate the light and the dark within us and move closer to inhabiting our essence. This *sūtra* stresses that we receive the gift of being truly ourselves through the grace of this power. The power is the force to battle not knowing. The process of integration and realization is teamwork between us and it. And this is the result of our learning outwards through *yama* and learning inwards through *niyama*.

When we hand over the old selves we constructed, we can step into being who we truly are. We can live in freedom from pain and conflict from that place of integrated being.

How can you accept yourself for the way you are?
How can you utilize a power that comes from this?
Can you begin to sense a direction of evolution in yourself? Is there a thread that could guide you?

Exercise for observing your attitudes in life

From now on, make it part of your daily practice to observe your behaviours and attitudes without criticism. Use the points above to investigate them. Do this exercise either at the beginning or towards the end of the day and reflect on an interaction you've had recently out in the world.

Observe the thoughts or feelings that came up for you, and whether that interaction made you more or less comfortable. What do you notice? Are your outward interactions smooth but your inner attitudes painful, for example? Or is it the other way round?

If you do this exercise regularly you will begin to notice patterns. Are you getting more or less comfortable in different areas of your life? Remember, it can be uncomfortable to investigate our behaviours, but the observation of them will support you to begin to change, so don't worry if you feel a little worse before you feel better. The key when you observe something is not to react. Is there more coherence in the way you feel about different aspects of your life? Is there less conflict with other people? Do disagreements get resolved faster? Do you see things more clearly?

If you're not sure, ask yourself more specific questions. You will probably know what sort of lines of inquiry will be most helpful in your case, but here are a few you could try:

1. When did I last have a disagreement with someone I love? How did I react at the time? How long did I hold on to it for? How do I see things now?

2. When have I apologized lately? Did I do it to avoid or to take responsibility? How did that feel?

3. When I experience feelings of anger or guilt or fear, what am I holding on to? Can I be honest and take responsibility for them?

4. Have any new emotions arisen that I don't understand and am trying to make sense of? Can I associate their appearance with a positive evolution in my understanding?
5. Is there a different way to tackle difficulties in my life?
6. How am I sleeping? Resting? Relaxing? How do I feel when I wake and when I go to sleep? Can I embrace flexibility in my approach to sleep and rest?

Group 14: Pitfalls, setbacks and how to deal with them

So, you are well on your way to incorporating yoga into your life. You're beginning to feel some benefits, to notice progress and to enjoy the exploration for its own sake. But then something knocks you off your path. Perhaps you get ill and are too poorly to practise. Or you get complacent, or lazy, or doubts set in. You forget that this is a lifelong learning (if you allow it to be) and you settle for having reached a particular plateau. Or life just gets too busy, or your spirits fall, you overindulge your senses with comforts and pleasures and you give in to the downward spiral for a while. However it happens, it isn't ideal when we lose our way, but it's certainly not a catastrophe. Treat yourself with compassion and just try again.

This group of *sūtra* looks at setbacks as forms of disconnection from the self. If yoga practice allows us to create a stronger link between different aspects of our selves, then impediments to practice take us further away from that integration and connection with the essence of who we are. We slip back into misunderstanding, or give in to our ego's whispering that we're pretty good at this yoga stuff now. These moments are just part of life. There is always help at hand.

Many setbacks; one solution (1.30)

There's no such thing as the perfect journey to being a yogi. Yoga, as we've already seen, is not a conveyor belt to enlightenment. You are going to have times in your life when you don't practise, when you can't be bothered, when you think there's nothing left to learn. Hopefully, you can bring clarity of vision to the situation as quickly and as gently as possible. That way the setbacks will be temporary and the journey will continue, enriched by what you've learned in the course of dealing with the obstacle.

This *sūtra* shows us that yoga practice is always the way to overcome whatever is blocking you. Too ill to do yoga? You can still meditate in your sick bed or do some very gentle movements and feel better. Feeling paralysed by indecision or doubt? If you were seeing clearly, you would realize that there is only ever one choice. In a hurry to move on to the next stage (whether of practice or of life)? Being in a rush is always a sign of an agitated mind. Slow down and connect to what's really going on right now. Got in the habit of relying on sensual pleasures or overstimulation, and feeling sluggish as a consequence? Turn off Netflix and do some simple breathing and postures instead. Feeling pleased with yourself, or wretched about yourself? Struggling to distinguish between who you can be and who you want to be? What you need, in all these situations, is your yoga practice to help.

Any of these blocks might stop us from continuing our journey if we let them, but the only way to figure them out and move through them is to view everything we're doing or experiencing as an experiment in practice. An inability to persevere can be fixed over time with attentive meditation. A sense of uncertainty can be relieved through breathwork.

Life's setbacks and confusions are signs that our minds are not in a yoga state. They provide the opportunity for us to evolve. The quicker we can recognize them as the messengers they are, the quicker we can begin to move towards that yoga state of mind.

> *How can you keep checking in with yourself and not let things go? Can you view illness, laziness, doubt, haste, excessive indulgence, delusion, an inability to persevere, regression or apathy as an opportunity to evolve?*

Learn your warning signs (1.31)

Wouldn't it be great if life came with an equivalent of those warning signs on the motorway that flash out, 'Slow down – incident ahead'? Actually, in some situations, life does. Long before a crisis, our minds and bodies will be sending us warnings. It's our job to pay attention, spot them and then act on them.

If you regularly experience emotional distress, for example, especially if it's consistently triggered by a particular person or situation, that's a big, fat warning sign. Same thing with negative thinking or agitated physiology, such as a twitch in your eye, palpitations or constipation. If you notice that you're holding on to your breath or that you feel you never quite breathe out fully, that's another one. If your mind is restless and you find it difficult to switch off to sleep or settle down to concentrate . . . guess what? More warnings. These signals are flashing orange, trying to alert you to the fact there's an obstacle in the road up ahead and you need to slow down to meet it.

They are also signalling that you've got an opportunity coming up, because on the flip side of every obstacle is an opportunity to change course. Our issues are not just problems to be solved. They are far more positive than that. When we learn how to recognize the help our minds and bodies are continually offering us, it becomes much easier to stay on a path away from suffering and towards our true selves.

Next time you notice one of your warning signs, can you commit to investigating? Can you begin to plan a different action from the one you usually take?

Find the thing that works for you, and stick at it (1.32)

It's safe to say that yoga is definitely my thing. I recognize that I am unusually single-minded in my practice, and that most people – even those for whom yoga is an important part of life – take a more magpie-like approach. They gather useful pieces of advice about their wellbeing, fitness and relationships from all kinds of sources. This tactic works for some people some of the time, but it isn't always great for everyone. Sometimes, it's better to find one trusted approach that works well for you, and just keep plugging away.

The problem is, most of us get more excited by new objects, people and ideas than we do by the familiar. Open-minded curiosity can never be a bad thing, but it's not always helpful, when we come up against an obstacle, to assume that we need to find a new way to tackle it. The fact that we've hit a glitch doesn't necessarily mean that we're on the wrong path. If we never persist, we never master a skill or build our confidence. We can end up trapped in a desiring mindset where we are led by what we want – rather than recognizing what we need. And what we want is often a quick fix for a problem, whereas what we need is sustained practice to clarify our understanding and keep making slow but steady progress.

I hope you are discovering that the thing that works for you is yoga. But if yoga is not your thing, by all means go on searching. Just try to ensure you're looking for what you need rather than what you want.

Are you able to resist the lure of novelty and reframe consistency as rewarding? To see consistent regular practice as an opportunity, not a chore?

Cultivate a peaceful mind for a peaceful life (1.33)

This *sūtra* is a powerful practical tool that makes it easier to maintain balance and boundaries in all your relationships, including the one you have with yourself. It describes four measures for a peaceful mind: friendliness, compassion, appreciation of what we perceive as positive and equanimity about what we perceive as negative. It also provides a marker for how your own personal evolution is going.

When our hearts are open and our minds are stable, these qualities flow and we naturally find it easier to have harmonious interactions with other people and with different aspects of ourselves. When they're not flowing, conflict is likely to result. Once we've noticed an uptick in conflict or discomfort, power struggles or indecision, we know we need to practise reacting with more of these four qualities of mind in order to get back to a peaceful state. This can't be forced. It's impossible and counterproductive to pretend to be cool about something that has, in fact, hurt you, for example. Faking equanimity in this way will only get you into more trouble.

Imagine that a friend has had a terrible year. They lost their job and split up with their partner. They've been behaving thoughtlessly for months now, draining your energy, borrowing money without returning it, demanding time and attention, never asking you how you are. How do you react? You value this person and don't want to fight, but you don't want things to remain as they are, either. You feel really sorry for them but increasingly irritated by them.

Experience has shown me that there is a process we must go through in response to any challenge or change in life. Unless we examine and manage our own feelings about events, using the four measures of gratitude, compassion, appreciation and equanimity, we won't attain genuine peace. In the end we'll bottle up our negative emotions and fake more 'acceptable' responses.

For example, it can be tempting to shoot straight for compassion for our annoying (if troubled) friend. 'They've had such an awful time,' we might say. And then try to convince ourselves that we're fine with the situation, that we just need to 'rise above it'. (Those of us who are heavily invested in believing that we are a 'nice' person are particularly likely to fall into this compassion trap.) But if you aim for equanimity and compassion without putting in the emotional work that's required to actually attain them, your mind will not be at peace. Conflict with your friend is inevitable – not because of what they have done or not done but because of what you have done, and not done.

The alternative is to absorb the lesson of this *sūtra*: our responses and reactions to life are under our control and will determine how easy or stressful we find it. Sometimes it's not our friend who should be our first port of call for compassion but ourselves. If you're hurt and angry, listen to yourself as you would a loved one. Offer comfort. Don't mistake this for self-pity – your self-compassion is a way to move into authentic compassion for your struggling friend.

These days, I aim to slow down my emotional processing enough to get to authentic appreciation for all my privileges and strokes of fortune. I aim for authentic compassion by listening, not taking sides and offering practical help to relieve suffering – my own as well as other people's. I aim to acknowledge and amplify compassionate acts wherever they are committed. I aim not to overreact to selfish or thoughtless acts. If I committed them, I take responsibility. If somebody else did, I take responsibility for my reaction. In this way I mostly avoid conflict. I also (mostly) avoid falling into the gratitude and compassion traps. My mind, like my life, is more peaceful as a result.

> *How do you act when other people are happy? Can you accept your own happiness? How do you react to somebody in pain? What about when you're in pain? Do you notice the good that others do? What do you do when you do good? Do you get caught up in the disrespect that you feel? How do you cope when you let others down? Having examined these, how could you navigate each of these feelings differently?*

Group 15: A question of faith

I've had many opportunities to observe that inspiration helps to change lives. Human beings need something to believe in, whether that's a god, a political cause or a set of personal values. Without some sort of belief system to put our faith in, we struggle to make life meaningful. Sometimes that struggle can make us truly miserable.

This group of *sūtra* explores yoga's relationship with spirituality and our relationship with what we believe in. It's a profound group of writings and can be read on so many different levels. As always, there's something for everyone here.

Some people see it as a discussion of how to relate to God, or to a higher state of consciousness. Other people see it as an exploration of the link between a teacher and a pupil, or a seeker and a guide. Perhaps it is about how we link with the universal wisdom that exists inside us, as it does within every individual.

For me, every *sūtra* – however I read it – encapsulates the idea that belief is an engine of change, both in my own life and in the world. What you choose to believe, and who you choose to follow, is profoundly important. Not every belief system is benign. If beliefs can bring about changes for the good, they can also spur people to acts of destruction.

Who will you pick as a success to emulate? How will you find your teachers? Are you open to the idea of receiving wisdom from unlikely sources? From a higher state of consciousness, however you define that? These *sūtra* show us different ways to think about our answers to these questions.

In search of your personal guide (1.23)

Yoga is not a religion. It doesn't talk about a god who created the world and it doesn't depend on a hierarchy of priests, imams or gurus. It is, however, inherently interested in spiritual matters. In this *sūtra* it introduces the concept of *Īśvara*, which translates as 'the one who carries power' but which in fact can take any form you choose to give it.

Can you imagine a figure of total trustworthiness? On a simple practical level, it could be the person who always has your back, who listens without judgement and offers you useful insights. So a personal mentor or a role model, perhaps. Or maybe it's a more abstract force for good. This might be a deity, or perhaps Nature. Maybe it's a system of thought that inspires and sustains people, and generates positive energy and compassion in the world.

This role model, guide, benign force or system, however you want to imagine it, is your own personal understanding of *Īśvara*. The *Yoga Sūtra* makes it plain that this entity, whatever it is, wants nothing from you. And the closer you come to it – through meditation – the closer you come to yoga.

You probably won't have much of an understanding of *Īśvara* yet, and that's absolutely fine. We're not defining anything here; we're just looking for ways to explore how you understand the powers that have made you uniquely *you*. This exploration takes place through meditation, practice and reflection. It takes time. A crucial aspect of your exploration will be looking for ways you can link with it, in order to get out of trouble and build success.

Where do you start? What do you or can you believe in that doesn't want anything from you – yet had your back? Can you begin to imagine, even if you only glimpse it, a figure of total support whose intention is simply to lift you up?

An ally in the quest to be comfortable with not knowing (1.24)

Yoga is a system for reducing the quantity of unknowns in our lives. It's the habit of trying to step back from our emotions and desires and assess what's really going on, with as much clear vision as we possibly can.

But even more fundamentally, yoga is a system for helping us accept that we will never get to 100 per cent clarity of understanding. Accepting this is a challenge, because not knowing what's going on, or what will happen, or why people behave as they do, or what something means, can make us feel horribly unsafe and uncomfortable. That's why we leap to find answers, tell stories and project our version of reality.

Īśvara is beyond all these strategies. It will hold you and support you to be OK with not knowing. This *sūtra* gives us an example (because we all need examples) of one aspect of this framework. It describes *Īśvara* as being beyond *kleśa*, so it contains no ego, feels no desire and no fear, has no attachments and is entirely comfortable with not knowing. It is available to be linked with, but seeks nothing from you and has no plans – either for you or for itself. It's an ally that cannot be corrupted. This is a radically challenging idea but a truly exciting one as well.

What can you observe about the intentions of your potential allies? Seek out people who do not have a strong agenda for you beyond supporting your growth. Don't forget to be an ally to others.

The source of all knowledge (1.25)

Here comes another way of thinking about *Īśvara*: as the source or seed of everything we know. This *sūtra* encourages you to explore what this source of knowledge might be like. Is it to be found outside us or inside us?

If it is outside, that puts it closer to the idea of a god, though perhaps not the kind of god most of us are familiar with. The *Yoga Sūtra* clarifies that, unlike the God of Christianity, Judaism and Islam, whatever this force or principle is, it is not omnipotent. As we saw in the previous *sūtra*, *Īśvara* is not all-powerful – in fact, it does not even take action itself. Now we see that neither is it all-knowing – rather, it is the source of all that is known.

If *Īśvara* is inside us, were we born with it or did we acquire it gradually?

I love that the *Yoga Sūtra* doesn't impose answers. It asks questions that allow us to glimpse the idea of limitless potential for knowledge. When I read this *sūtra* I always come away with more questions.

One question in particular seems to me to be most important here: What is there to know?

Timeless wisdom (1.26)

In many world religions God is thought to be eternal – a force without end. In this *sūtra*, *Īśvara* is presented as something completely *outside of* time. It has been making itself available for as long as human beings have needed guidance. It is timeless. It was the guide for our ancestors – for everyone who came before us – and will be for all those who come after us.

Īśvara is pointing the way beyond our obsession with time. So many of us feel time poor. We worry that we don't have enough time and fret about scheduling the time we do have. In yoga practice, many of us become obsessed with how long we sit for. If we sit for ten minutes we aspire to twenty. When we hear that a classmate sits for thirty minutes we immediately tell ourselves that we should be able to do the same.

Maybe we could think less about time in order to get beyond it? I believe there are places we can access that are beyond time's rules and obligations. They are the places that provide access to wisdom. This is why I suggest you don't set a timer for your yoga or meditation sessions. To constrict our practice with alarms is to encourage our obsession with measuring and 'making the most of' our time. It is a capitulation to chaos when we try to control it in this way. When we simply sit quietly, guided by our own internal clocks, responsive to what comes up, we are beginning to move towards timelessness. Two minutes or two hours, it really doesn't matter.

Do we have to put a timeframe
on everything? Why?

How should we link with Īśvara? (1.27)

This *sūtra* offers us some thoughts on how we might relate to the deeper consciousness, however we understand it. The instruction comes in two main parts and is very clear. Firstly, it is important to try, as far as we possibly can, to relate to *Īśvara* from a position that is not needy or desiring, ego-driven or inauthentic. The reason for this is simple: *Īśvara*'s immense powers will magnify our *kleśa* back at us. If we're looking for a sign that our practice is approved of, that's unlikely to end well. If we're straining to be 'holy', that's a warning sign. No one can eradicate all *kleśa*, of course (except *Īśvara* itself), but it's good to aim for humble, open inquiry in all your meditation on *Īśvara*.

The second suggestion is to use a sound that is sacred or special to us. This is most commonly realized as a spoken or chanted mantra that gathers our attention on understanding *Īśvara*. (If you've never used sounds before and don't know where to start, don't worry. There is guidance in the exercise at the end of this section.)

> *Can you begin to experiment with a tool that feels right for you? It could be connected to your external voice or your internal one. This will help you move beyond needing to be supplied with tools and build your confidence in finding your own.*

Your belief powers your connection to Īśvara (1.28)

There are no rules about how we should approach the deep consciousness, but this *sūtra* suggests that we practise with respect, patience and good faith, and that we practise consistently, using our voice tool frequently. When we take *Īśvara* seriously in this way, we are respecting the source of all the wisdom we ourselves contain. We're paying our dues to the unbroken chain of ancestors who came before us. We're also embodying self-respect. All of this combines to make our practice more powerful.

In order to cultivate the sincere commitment that sustains your connection to *Īśvara*, it can help to visualize it as a source of light that is both radiant and grounded. The image is less important than the feeling it conjures up in you. Remember that *Īśvara* always magnifies what you bring to it, so check your motivation and cultivate curiosity, friendliness and patience as you visualize.

> *What happens if you commit to opening up to* Īśvara *every day for a week? Even a minute of open-hearted reflection is enough. Choose to explore and follow your own directions.*

Align with Īśvara *and supercharge your practice* (1.29)

This *sūtra* tells us that if we work with *Īśvara*, however we understand it, its force becomes available to us. It promises two outcomes of this alignment. Firstly, our understanding of our selves will increase. Secondly, we will feel *Īśvara* working with us to reduce obstacles in our lives.

In these *sūtra* we are invited to create our own understanding of what *Īśvara* means to us. The text offers us pointers and asks us to consider some possibilities without any restrictions or demands. There is complete freedom here, but that poses its own challenges. Where do we even begin?

I like to start with questions. Whom do I admire and why? What do I find meaningful, moving, important? How can I get closer to those people and ideas? And what connection do they have with the lessons I need to learn?

Exercise for deepening your understanding of *Īśvara*

This is really more of an inquiry than an exercise. Here are some thoughts on how you might begin your personal investigation into *Īśvara*.

1. The first (and in some ways the most difficult) stage is to open up to the idea that a link with *Īśvara* is possible. It can be a stretch of the imagination to envisage being in contact with such a powerful and mysterious force, to be held by and to hold something full of light, and in a light way. It's a challenge to imagine entering into such a relationship. Is it within you? Is it something outside you? Is it both?
2. Thinking in abstract terms like this is hard for most of us, so focusing on concrete examples can help us to

do this work of imagination and trust building. Can you think of any people whose values and behaviour you admire? They might be a historical figure such as Nelson Mandela or a trusted friend or family member. What about places that console you or restore your energy, such as a favourite spot in the local woodland or in the mountains?

3. For some of us, this something greater than us is clearly God.
4. It doesn't really matter what you choose to meditate on as you explore the idea of a greater power and investigate how you could relate to it. The important thing is just to mull these ideas over. Sit in meditation and set your intention to let your thoughts roam and your feelings arise.
5. Your investigation will be open-ended and will probably involve many, many meditation sessions on a range of different potential sources of wisdom and support. Look to view all this as an interesting part of the process. There are no right or wrong answers. The only purpose is to investigate whether this more spiritual aspect of yoga is yet meaningful for you.
6. You will know that you're on the right track when you start to feel calmer and more secure during those times when you're looking for answers to life's inevitable questions. This is how I feel when I link with my yoga teacher, whether through conversation or in recollection or imagination. I feel more

confident about my beliefs and choices, and I feel somehow better – more hopeful and purposeful – about myself and the world. The connection I feel then goes beyond language. It's as if I'm able to hear a sacred sound. Perhaps it's his voice I hear, or perhaps it's my own inner voice. Whatever it is, I feel lighter.

Can you learn to stop overlaying the quiet inner voice with all the shouty outer voices?

Group 16: Yoga = meditation by any other name

In this group of *sūtra*, the final group we'll be looking at, we are examining the process of deepening our meditation. All yoga practice can be understood as meditation, and as we practise, we get more skilled at refining our meditation for better results. We're always aiming to experiment with and refine our interactions in life by using the eight components of yoga, learning from our attitudes to our environment (which includes other people) and to ourselves. We typically begin our work with postures and experiment with breathing and detaching from unhelpful habits. We begin to be aware of our relationships. Then we can start to move towards the trickier elements: cultivating an ability to direct our minds and focus, interacting simply and directly with what we're trying to understand and – eventually – integrating that object into our understanding. When you attain this objective, you will have turned your whole life into a meditative practice, living the practice of yoga with every step and every breath.

For me, the mechanism that underpins meditation is my mind's ability to focus on an object and then let go, focus and let go, over and over again, as smoothly as possible. 'Focus' describes that link between the conscious part of the mind – the perceiving element – and the object it perceives. In meditation, we focus on something and form a link with it. Some time later, we release our focus and do something else. It's like a plane taking off, flying for a while and then landing. The mark of a good pilot is to ensure that the take-off and landing are as smooth as possible. Think of your meditation practice as piloting your mind – it's the transitions into and out of meditation where we need to pay most attention, especially as a beginner. Don't worry how long you're flying for in between, just aim to get comfortable at treating meditation as a matter of picking up an object and putting it down: focus and release, like breathing in and out . . .

What will you choose to link with? (1.41)

All meditation (all thought, all action, all feeling) begins with a link between the part of the mind that is doing the perceiving and that which it perceives. When we begin yoga or sit down to meditate, our minds search for something to focus on: 'What's the instructor asking me to do? Is the next move a backwards lunge? I can't remember!' Or, 'Shall I do a loving-kindness meditation? That will give me a focus. But shouldn't I be clearing all my thoughts? I can't do it!' Our minds could pick virtually anything to focus on in any given situation, but typically (and unhelpfully) they tend to choose items such as those I've described here.

This is all entirely normal; it's just what minds do. The important thing is to realize that their attention magnifies the power of whatever it is they grasp – which can be helpful or very unhelpful. If our mind focuses on a criticism, for example, whether it's our inner critic calling us useless or our conscience berating us for telling a lie, the wounding power of the insult or the guilt and shame generated by the lie will grow in size. The consequences of focusing on something negative are always bad. If, instead, we can grasp on to a self-compassionate sense that we are doing our best and will have another go, we increase our chance of success.

What you choose to link with is under your control. Your mind is only as sticky as you allow it to be. Watch out for excuses along the lines of, 'I'm ADHD, I can't meditate.' You can; you just need more tools and you need to put them together in the right way for your mind. It will take practice, but get in the habit of assessing whether or not your focus is on something useful and worthwhile. Our best course of action, especially as beginner meditators/practitioners, is to bring awareness to what we are linking with. The mind takes on the colour of its surroundings, so try to ensure you're colouring it with things that will make it more powerful. Meditation is simply linking your mind to something. It is not out of reach for any of us and we don't need a special mind to do it.

Your mind can hold on to anything. It tells countless stories every day. How can you reduce your mental activities and improve your mind? Can you embrace the idea that your mind is powerful enough to do anything? How does your mind take the colour of its surroundings? How does the memory of what's come earlier in the day influence your involvement in what you're doing now? Can you begin to channel some of that incredible power in a direction you want?

In meditation, you get what you give (1.42)

Once you've understood that you are in control of what you focus on, you're all set to start working with the bad news that most of us, most of the time, are focused on the wrong things. As we saw in the example above, if you link with a negative emotion, you magnify it. If you link with a painful memory or a greedy fantasy, guess what? You're making it more powerful.

When we start out in meditation, it is inevitable that we link with low-level material objects we can perceive easily and that our meditations are tainted with loads of memory and imagination. Within the first stages of meditation there is contamination of words, meanings and knowledge. We just don't yet have the skills to see clearly and choose in a controlled way. It's important to recognize that none of us can bypass this stage. We all have to learn by going through it.

Imagine you are a new parent and your focus is naturally on your newborn. You're full of love for your child, excited to know them, but you're also nervous as hell. A new parent, depending on their personality type and experiences, might focus on their terror that something will happen to their baby, rather than their wonder at the baby's perfection or their deep tenderness and impulse to care for them. This is normal, natural, and as you get more experienced at living with your baby, you get more skilled at choosing to focus on joy and wonder rather than anxiety and fear. But you have to go through those first sleepless nights when you compulsively check on your baby's breathing. Only that way can you train your mind to focus its energy elsewhere.

It's the same with meditation, yoga, all of life. You can choose what you link with. In first-level meditation you will choose the wrong thing, unable to resist the power of ego, fear or desire that pulls you to link with something unhelpful. Don't berate yourself; just keep practising.

What will you choose to link with when you meditate today? What refuge or support will keep your mind focused? Your body? Your breath? A sound? An image? How can you recognize your identifications in this meditative interaction? What about your memories? And your imagination?

Practice brings the link into focus (1.43)

As you get more experienced in meditation, you will find it easier to turn away from painful feelings brought up by your memory or unreal feelings conjured up by your imagination. You will find it easier to create a link with something, and realize that the link itself is simple and good.

In the example of our new parent, they might begin to be able to enjoy the moment of interaction with their baby without any interference from fear or neediness. They are linked solely with the reality of their baby in this moment. The link between them is material, sensory and enveloping, and very real to the two parties who experience it, both of whom are communicating with one another via this link. All identities and knowledge have disappeared; there is just this link.

This next-level meditation can be a beautiful and rewarding experience, and it serves the immensely useful function of drawing our attention to itself so that we can grasp its radiant quality.

When keeping the mind focused, how can you evolve it so that your identifications disappear? What's left for you? Enjoy these moments of clarity, however fleeting and infrequent. Look not to hang on to them or seek them out; just appreciate them when they arrive and trust that there will be more.

Meditation becomes a dance of energy (1.44)

This *sūtra* develops the exploration of how our meditation becomes a more profound and rewarding practice. If we imagine our parent and newborn, enveloped in the experience of their meditative link, we can see that the mutual exchange of energy will deepen over time. As the parent smiles at the baby, the baby begins to smile back. The link operates like a mirror. It's deeper and more subtle.

For the parent there are still traces of memory and imagination impinging on the moment, but they have softened. Rather than being swept away when they suddenly remember a distressing story about a friend's baby who became seriously ill, for example, the parent experiences memory in short bursts that do not break the link with their child. The enveloping experience becomes golden and precious as the two of them send the energy of their minds back and forth, nourishing each other with a sustaining and present awareness.

Once we reach this stage of fluidity, the rewards of meditation are making themselves very obvious. Our awareness is such that the edge comes off life's surprises. Our ability to be present, be aware, be stable, be comfortable, be positive and be compassionate are all hugely increased.

Why is it that often, when we reach this point of ease, we freak out and try to control what we're focusing on? The trouble is that the beginner meditator's mind can't handle the intensity of such success. Negative associations or bad memories surge up to take advantage of our wobble. Call it 'revenge of the issues'. This is very common, so don't let it get you down.

What subtle quality or concept will you choose to focus on? Love? Peace? Space? Receiving? Giving? What comes up for you? When working with a subtle quality, if any issue arises then return to your starting point, no matter how insignificant you feel it is.

Let everything come to the surface (1.45)

Intermediate meditators experience greater clarity, comfort and stability. Having understood that what we link with becomes more powerful, both in itself and in us, and having got better at directing our energy to link with beneficial objects, we are ready to work with the feelings, thoughts and memories that come up for us.

When we sit in meditation, stuff comes up from our depths. This *sūtra* reminds us that everything deep within our minds must and will play out upon its surface. The subtle aspect of who we are must be manifest. We cannot ignore or outrun who we truly are, because our surface is always the expression of what's underneath. In the end, pretending to be something we're not is unsustainable. We will pay the price in an unquiet mind.

I love this *sūtra*, which is a reminder not to try to ignore what we'd rather not face. Understand that you can meditate for years and years and there is always something to discover the further we go. By doing our practice we develop the mind's ability to link with any and every thing it finds in its own depths. We are settling into our own authenticity. When the mind is stable and comfortable enough to form nourishing links, it can allow itself to be a seamless whole, without fear or shame or pride. With such integration comes freedom. It's as if each situation we find ourselves in is new again. So refreshing!

> *Do you think you have truly understood something? Or do you feel that you can remain open to discovering more? Can you practise taking responsibility for whatever comes to the surface, rather than wishing it away? Don't deny it or label it and don't hold on to it tightly. Learn from it.*

Meditation is the process, not the result (1.46)

This is a lovely and simple line that returns us to the image of a seed being the starting point for meditation, as it is for knowledge. None of us can magic up a peaceful mind – or a troubled one, come to that – out of nowhere. Every meditative state, whether low-level on a painful material object or super high-level, begins with a seed and then develops over time and with practice.

What do you choose to link to? If you can create a meditative link with an object that sustains and nourishes you, you will be able to sit for as long as needs be, even in the middle of chaos.

Be aware that you might need to update what you link with. A seed grows into a tree. Remember that in order to stay stable you have to respond to constant changes by adapting yourself.

See yourself in the serene spot (1.47)

This *sūtra* conjures up a picture of how life might look when we are truly comfortable with ourselves. Through meditation it encourages us to be very good at doing something. At this level of practice, we are able to see life's chaos very clearly and be OK with it. We do not choose to link with it but we acknowledge its reality. Instead, we focus on serenity, the space beyond chaos. Linking with that, we create an energetic envelope that allows us to know our own consciousness fully. It's like an expression of pure creativity that comes from our hearts and just flows through you without any effort. You just know and trust that wisdom. It's the reward for all that practice. It's living with the benefits of genuine serenity, stability and clarity.

What is it that you are very good at? Can you let it flow? Can you imagine yourself as someone who has been meditating for ten years? What comes up as you investigate this thought?

Truth is a by-product of wisdom (1.48)

Here's another *sūtra* that helps us to understand how meditation operates. When we're working at our highest level, our practice generates truth, which is the full alignment between our perspective and relationship on our selves and on the world. We perceive reality as much as possible as it is and expose our full genuine personality.

I find it really interesting that the *Yoga Sūtra* talks about truth as the by-product of a long and potentially arduous process of self-exploration, refining our capacity to be honest to and about ourselves.

'Truth' is a slippery category in our world. Sometimes it seems to mean nothing more than 'my version of events'. But as I hope you've understood by now, our minds are always clouded by ignorance (not knowing), desire (the products of ego), fear and the many other elements of *kleśa* that stop us from being able to see clearly or explain honestly.

This *sūtra* promises that the truth that will emerge when we've been doing our work will look and feel very different from the truth we asserted before we began. There's a happy, real and serene quality to it. Truth is never an argument, or an attempt to persuade. It is peace. It is the capacity to listen deeply in order to understand fully.

Can you experiment with approaching each day as either a blank or a possibility? Can you practise the readiness that allows you to take each day lightly, in full awareness that the nature of plans is that they change? Can you allow yourself to expose your genuine personality?

The highest knowledge is closer than you think (1.49)

If you're feeling nervous about all this talk of truth and higher knowledge, this *sūtra* arrives just in time to reassure you.

When we meditate skilfully, openly, serenely, we know things in a powerful and instinctive way. This sort of knowledge is not what we learn from our elders or peers, or in school. It is not even what we learn from careful observation of our own experience. It's closer to a form of very deep intuition.

Most of us will have experienced, at some point in our lives, a certainty that seems to arrive not via our brain's intellectual capacities but from deep inside us, or even from outside us. Gut instinct. A flash of insight. The sudden sense of knowing another person intimately that overtakes us when we're falling in love. There are many ways that human beings come to know things. High-level meditation is another of them.

Most of us have been taught to distrust these alternative ways of knowing. We worry that they might lead us astray. We worry they could come from unreliable emotions. We think they might be delusions. We jump away from such moments of insight and back into familiar ways of thinking, at which point the link is broken and we lose that knowledge.

In meditation, we learn to be comfortable in such moments and focus on them with loving, inquiring trust rather than fear or doubt. This can feel like a revelation or a deep sense of security. You don't have to be enlightened to experience it; you just have to be a dedicated meditator, prepared to put some time in.

How can you be open to a different way of thinking? How can you be open to trusting the deeper feeling that's beyond words more?

The possibility to genuinely change our habits (1.50)

When we are in touch with a truth that comes from a higher knowledge and can trust its insights, a different way of living becomes possible. In order to grasp this moment of potential we have trained our minds to be stable in the midst of chaos. We have fully integrated the habit of making small tweaks to our ways of thinking in order to maintain stability amid constant change. We understand that success is a small adjustment, not a reinvention.

This *sūtra* is a huge and beautiful promise. It says that when we trust in the truth that emerges in these moments of insight, anything is possible. True change is possible with a meditative mind. The change you are working towards is yours to be embodied. You are who you are, and you are beautiful. Your potential is infinite.

Can you prioritize getting to a point of stability in order to change things, rather than changing things to try and find stability? How can you be open to the possibility of changing your patterns from this place?

Always leave a door open (1.51)

True meditation is so powerful that anything is possible. It creates a portal to taking our practice even higher. It holds out as an evolution the prospect of being able to meditate on absolutely nothing at all – no object or focus required. No dividing lines between you, your mind and the object of your meditation; between the perceiver, what's doing the perceiving and the perceived. If any of us are lucky enough to experience this in our lifetime, this is the place of true peace.

I haven't met anyone who claims to have used this methodology successfully – though for me the important message is to keep a door open. You never know. The fact that we haven't yet got there is not a cause for regret or blame but a reason to get excited by the promise of continual evolution.

> *How can you leave the door open for your evolution? How can you keep going even after you think you've got there?*

Loop back and take another journey . . .

I invite you to be open to all of this infinite potential as a real possibility for you. Take it with you as you end one cycle of learning and consider where to go next. Reading the *Yoga Sūtra* again will show you many more insights. You could restart the pathway we have already picked out, back on page 29 of this book, at *sūtra* 2.46. If you re-read that path with different eyes, I guarantee that many new ideas will come to you. Or you could pick a different starting point – Group 10 or Group 13, wherever you choose – begin there and cycle through the pages that way. You could, if you wished, read the first two chapters of the *Yoga Sūtra* in sequence. Or in reverse. It's all waiting for you, printed at the back of the book.

I invite you to step through the portal and see what you find. You are open to much more intuitive learning and much deeper meditation than you perhaps realize. We all are. So please, keep on journeying into yoga.

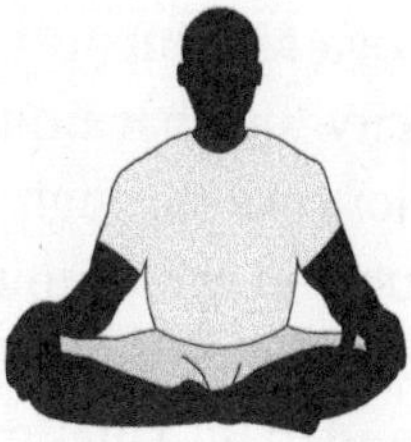

5. *How to Extend Your Yoga Journey*

Your introduction to yoga as a support system for living with more clarity, authenticity and harmony is complete. I hope that you've found this journey through the ancient wisdom of the *Yoga Sūtra* rewarding and eye-opening. As you've probably realized by now, yoga as a philosophy for life is a big subject, one that can easily expand to fill a lifetime. It's as adaptable and flexible as you are and, if you can sustain your practice, it will reward your attention in so many ways.

So where to next, on your unique yoga journey? This final chapter of the book opens with thoughts on keeping your practice going, because without consistency, progress in any direction is impossible. Then it offers suggestions for a number of different paths you could explore. They are not mutually exclusive, nor do you have to follow any of them – you might already have a clear sense of how to keep moving on your path towards yoga. There's a whole universe of exploration available to you. Where will you choose to go?

First, sustain your practice

I very much hope that you're excited and curious about having yoga in your life, but experience has shown me that it can be hard to keep practising when that initial excitement wears off, as it inevitably does. Realistic expectations are essential to keeping up your engagement and motivation. This is a long game. If you're sprinting for the next revelation, you're only running faster towards the limbo of disappointment.

Limbo is what I call that period of weary trudging through a kind of mental no man's land that happens to all of us who are on a path towards yoga, when it feels as if we're stuck on a plateau and nothing is happening. The days when your yoga practice never failed to empower you with new insights are long gone. You start to feel that wherever you've reached is as far as you can go.

This is the moment when you might want to give up on yoga and try something else. I urge you to disengage from that impulse and just keep going. So long as you keep practising and ignore the mirages of supposedly better alternatives, yoga will move you on towards the limit of what you personally are capable of. And at some point, you will realize that whatever notion of progress you were aiming for was just another mirage and that your daily practice has brought you further than you could ever have imagined when you started out. The no man's land you're trapped in dissolves around you, and you see that it was never a reality.

Now you're in a different place, going through rapid growth towards the very best that you can be, physically, emotionally, energetically. After that comes a maintenance phase, in which you practise to conserve all the gains you've made. Your daily practice allows you to manage the effects of ageing, to avoid catastrophizing about it and to grow in wisdom. For many of us there eventually comes a phase when we withdraw somewhat from the busy demands of the world and turn towards appreciation, creativity, contemplation.

None of these phases is inevitable or necessary but I have seen them all happen many times, so I'm outlining them to you as one example of the way a yoga practice can develop over a lifetime.

A long-term yoga practice protects your ability to live your life in the way you choose, and to maintain a coherent link between how you feel inside and outside your body. The key elements to cultivate are curiosity, patience and consistency. Embrace the notion of progress as a shuffling forward in tiny steps, and trust to that momentum.

Yoga in times of grief and loss

Hospices are some of the most amazing places I've ever worked in. Their focus is on supporting people with terminal illness to live the best possible life in the short time they have left. Yoga therapy might be offered alongside palliative care, including pain relief, other complementary therapies such as aromatherapy and massage, as well as gardening, entertainments, great food and comfortable spaces for a person's family and friends to be with them. Contrary to what you might imagine, hospices are peaceful and serene, full of light and laughter. There is, of course, distress and sadness, but there's also a profound sense that everyone is living right in the moment, appreciating what's still good and important, and choosing to focus on those things.

The truth is that we all have choices about what to connect with at every moment. If we can strengthen our capacity to link with objects that are beneficial for us when times are good, we are building our capacity to protect our minds and spirits, even when we are faced with the most devastating losses. Yoga therapy cannot 'cure' the heartbreak experienced by someone facing the certainty that they will soon die, or by that person's loved ones when it comes to pass. There is no remedy for pain of that kind. But yoga *can* be a catalyst for healing from even devastating loss. When we link with our fear, anger or despair, either by denying it or dwelling in it, we make it stronger. If, on the other hand, we open up to those feelings by accepting them, allowing them to come up and be felt in the knowledge that they will pass, we are connecting with our full humanity.

I particularly remember one woman I met while I was working in the hospice. She was coming every day to visit her husband, who was dying of pancreatic cancer. I was running sessions with patients and with the palliative-care nurses, who were desperately vulnerable to emotional and physical burnout. During a break, I got talking to this lady. She was struggling to stay connected with her husband because her grief was overwhelming, which was adding to her distress because she didn't want to miss a second of the time she had left with him. When I suggested she might benefit from some simple breathing work combined with postures, for just ten minutes at a time, she agreed to try. I hoped that it would allow her a tiny break from her pain, and it did seem to help. She was able to look after herself by dropping into a moment of peace when she needed to.

Yoga cannot take away the pain of loss, but what it can do is give us a moment of respite. Sometimes, that moment is the difference between being able to carry on and collapsing.

During the lockdowns that were imposed to contain the Covid pandemic, I did a lot of work with people using Zoom. Many of them were struggling with a sense of frustration or even despair about the loss of freedom, connection with loved ones, income, opportunity and so many other things besides. They were grieving for this loss in ways that were making them unwell.

One man I spoke with every week was obsessed with the question of when he would be able to 'get back to normal'. He was torturing himself with this question, to which nobody knew the answer, and could not make any kind of peace with not knowing. He was very distressed by a number of traumatic losses that had occurred in the previous few years, including the death of his mother and his own struggle with cancer. The pandemic had been the final blow to his resilience and he was suffering terribly with anxiety.

We worked together to look more attentively at the reality of his situation. He was convinced that the problem was lock-down and he was afraid that his marriage was not strong enough to survive it. It gradually became apparent that he had not released his emotions around his previous losses. We asked those fundamental questions 'What's really going on here?' and 'What's making me uncomfortable?' over and over again.

Alongside this investigation I showed him ways to relieve his distress with breathing exercises like the one on page 109 and the meditation for disengaging with insomnia on page 167. I gave him a wide variety of exercises and tools, including mantras and meditations, because his mind was very restless and I could see he would benefit from variety.

As he grew less anxious, he began to see more clearly. He was able to move towards an acceptance of uncertainty and he built up his belief that he could and would survive this experience. When he was reasonably stable, we were able to start discussing the *Yoga Sūtra*'s teachings around loss and grief in the context of change and volatility. He saw for himself that the lines in the sand he had been drawing ('Life must get back to normal otherwise I can't cope') were neither true nor helpful. He was able to acknowledge the reality of the profound losses imposed by lockdown, as well as his mother's death and his own illness, without his mind collapsing into them.

I was so pleased to be able to help, and I know that we can all learn to help ourselves in this way, even in a crisis, if we apply ourselves. It is much easier to do this if we have already taught ourselves to sit in the middle of everyday chaos. I practise yoga in good times so that when the bad times arrive, I will still be able to.

Yoga during illness: as complement to conventional healthcare

I know, from years of working as a yoga therapist alongside doctors in hospices and clinics, that yoga and Western medicine are both deeply powerful and absolutely complementary. When a client comes to me with symptoms I always urge them to get every conventional test going. The more information, the better. I work alongside doctors who feel the same way about yoga, who see it as a powerful tool that complements their own work.

Yoga's approach to mental and physical wellness works hand in hand with Āyurveda, the ancient Indian understanding of health and medicine. Yoga and Āyurveda maintain that both body and mind process the inputs they receive, keeping some elements and expelling others on the way. Our bodies consume food and liquid and then at each level make decisions about what to extract for their nutritional value, what to pass on to the next physiological process and what to excrete. Sometimes this process doesn't always work. Sometimes nutrition gets stuck at a relatively superficial level, leaving us undernourished deep within our system. Sometimes we eliminate what we should keep. Sometimes we can't metabolize or assimilate.

As with our bodies, so with our minds: we are constantly taking in, passing on and letting go of information. There must be effective communication between every level of the system for it to work well. The brain acquires information via the sensory organs. Some of that information is incorporated into its working knowledge, some it files for easy access and some it deposits in the deepest storeroom of its subconscious. If this process is obstructed by an emotional block, or we are so full and overwhelmed that our minds cannot absorb what they are receiving and simply rush to eliminate it, then the ecosystem that is our selves – those body-mind-heart-spirit organisms we call home – will become *dis*-eased.

Some followers of yoga maintain that all illness is the result of emotional blockage. This is too simplistic for me, but it's certainly true that yoga emphasizes the interlinked nature of the human organism. It insists that a blockage in processing in one area will have a knock-on effect everywhere. This model helps to explain why somebody with unprocessed grief from a bereavement many years ago might develop digestive problems, or a person who is dealing with fatigue can be helped to feel better by releasing the anger they feel towards their symptoms. If we work with the natural flow of our organisms' processing, our interventions to tackle the disease are likely to produce better results.

According to Āyurveda, everything in the world – including the human organism – is made up of five elements: ether, air, fire, water and earth. These elements combine to be summarized as three distinct bodily constitutions or humours – *vāta*, *pitta* and *kapha*. Each of these is associated with certain functions, characteristics, traits and maladies. Every individual's constitution is unique, determined by the particular ratios of bodily humours within their system. For most people, one or two dominate. Very few have all three.

Certain constitutions are prone to certain conditions, but as well as natural susceptibility there is also a natural resilience. Each person's expression of their constitution is also constantly changing, whether as a result of changes in the environment, ageing, biological events such as pregnancy and menopause, the impact of stress or illness or a change in diet.

Yoga is tortoise-style healing. If we use the correct tool targeted in a good way it can release us from unpleasant symptoms if we give it enough time to work, but it is the absolute opposite of a pill to pop. Yoga can also *relieve* our discomfort while we're doing the long-term work of *releasing* it. This is especially true if we practise yoga for healing as a way of life rather than a one-off treatment.

There will be many factors that contribute to you feeling unwell. In order to understand where your symptoms come from, it can help to ask yourself questions about your personal history, daily habits, diet, relationships: everything. How do you process thoughts and emotions? How does your body respond to food and movement? How do you react to stressors and temptations, pleasures and pains?

When we first sit down to examine how we process what our bodies and minds are taking in, it can feel a little daunting. We feel like detectives investigating our own lives. We must observe how our issues change from day to day and month to month. We must listen to how our stories about them change, too. What's feeling better this week? What's feeling worse?

This approach is highly nuanced. Effective diagnosis and treatment are not achievable for an untrained person working alone; most often they require a collaboration between patient and doctor. But we can all benefit from deepening our understanding of how we process everything we take in. Over time, we will build a clearer understanding of the root of our trouble.

One very important piece of general advice is not to try to fix all your problems at once, and not to try all possible strategies at the same time. If you do, you'll get overwhelmed and you won't be certain what's helping and what's not. Remember, the basis of using yoga to relieve your symptoms is to observe what triggers them and what relieves them. You will find it easier to do this one symptom at a time. So, please, try to identify your priority concern and consider what feels like a realistic aim for improvement. Step back and sanity-check your story around your symptoms, your emotions and your worries. Then have another look at your priority, in case it's changed.

It's helpful to remind ourselves of first principles. Yoga teaches us that we often do not see clearly. Don't be too quick to assume that you know what's causing your symptoms. Keep a diary to track them and, above all, keep an open mind.

Yoga as the foundation of a life of service or activism

All spiritual and many philosophical and political traditions stress the importance of setting aside our egos and thinking of what other people need, and how we might be able to provide it. The values of generosity, community and service are very strong in many cultures, even where there is no religious dimension, and yoga is no exception. In our own secular society, science has shown that human beings (like all social animals) generally struggle in isolation, and neuroscience has shown that (perhaps as a consequence) we're hardwired to be altruistic and compassionate. On some level, most of us know that life has more meaning, and is more rewarding, when we live from a mindset of 'we' rather than 'I'.

As we've seen many times in the first two chapters of the *Yoga Sūtra*, yoga is very concerned with living a life that's faithful to our own values while always being considerate of others. The text shows us over and over again that we must respect other people's integrity by being aware of what they think and how they feel, and adapt our own actions with that in mind. In this way, the empathy and patience that are the very foundations of service are woven throughout the sections of the *Yoga Sūtra* that we've looked at.

Yoga as a spiritual practice

Yoga can be deeply satisfying on a spiritual level. I hope our exploration of the *sūtra* about linking with the idea of something powerful or higher has given you a starting point for extending your journey in this direction. I would definitely recommend that you study the whole text of the *Yoga Sūtra* if you are interested in the more spiritual side of yoga. There are countless books about yoga and spirituality or esoteric thinking. Have a look at the short reading list at the back of this book for some of my favourites.

The wonder of yoga's understanding of spiritual matters is that it is so practical and realistic. Yoga has always felt to me like a form of spiritual philosophy for people who live in the real world. I hope that you have found many places in this book where your understanding of how to live in the world with grace and serenity has been deepened. Yoga supports everyday contemplation for people who want to connect with others as well as themselves. In this sense I find it a particularly great resource for people whose spiritual practice includes service to others, activism, caring, community work or simply being a great friend.

Yoga for your one precious life

I'd like to finish with some reminders – a sort of checklist for a yoga life.

- Firstly, remember that you have everything you need within you already; you just have to unpack it. This is liberating because it means you do not need to depend on what other people give you. You can be free just to relate to them.
- Do remember that there are two sides to everything: the dark and the light. This includes yourself. Embrace both.
- Your personal evolution (like everybody else's) is a never-ending story. There is huge comfort and wisdom in this idea. It's the opposite of perfection or culmination.
- If you fall, pick yourself up, go back to where you were and look not to make the same mistake again.
- Remember that your energy and attention will nourish whatever you direct them towards – positive or negative. Make sure you're feeding trust and confidence rather than fear. What might happen if you were to put the same amount of energy into your meditation practice as you do into your worries and resentments?

- Avoid over-involvement with inherited traumas that have been passed on by your parents or from your family's past. You can still break the chains of transmission by keeping an eye on the anger you learned from your father, for example, without feeding it in your own life with too much attention.
- Try to be realistic about who you think you are, who you want to be and who you really are on any given day. They won't be three identical versions of yourself, and that's OK.
- Beware the seductive power of the idea of cause and effect. Most change is not as simple as an on/off switch. The change that occurs in yoga is most definitely not like that. Sometimes you might feel that you've had a moment of revelatory understanding or development and that can feel glorious, until you lose it again. Most of the change in yoga comes as a result of patient shuffling forward on slippery ground. You can go a long way like this. As far as you wish.
- What's your priority in life? Shuffle in that direction.
- If in doubt, sit down, breathe and see what happens.

Thank you for staying with me. I hope you're feeling more serene and more stable in the face of life's chaos. I invite you to keep practising; I truly hope you will. And remember, the *Yoga Sūtra* will keep feeding you its wisdom for as long as you keep reading.

Appendix I: Chapter One of the Yoga Sūtra

atha – now, *samādhi* – integration, *pādaḥ* – chapter

1.1 *atha* – now, *yoga* – yoga, *anuśāsanam* – the teaching

1.2 *yogaḥ* – yoga, *citta* – mind, *vṛtti* – activities, *nirodhaḥ* – ability to envelop

1.3 *tadā* – then, *draṣṭuḥ* – the perceiver, *svarūpe* – in its own form, *avasthānam* – established

1.4 *vṛtti* – activities of the mind, *sārūpyam* – identification, *itaratra* – elsewhere

1.5 *vṛttayaḥ* – the activities of the mind, *pañcatayyaḥ* – five kinds, *kliṣṭā* – cause of hurt, *akliṣṭāḥ* – not producing hurt

1.6 *pramāṇa* – correct comprehension, *viparyaya* – misunderstanding, *vikalpa* – imagination, *nidrā* – sleep, *smṛtayaḥ* – memory

1.7 *pratyakṣa* – direct experience, *anumāna* – reflective inference, *āgamāḥ* – credible reference, *pramāṇāni* – correct comprehension

1.8 *viparyayo* – misunderstanding, *mithyā* – false, *jñānam* – knowledge, *atadrūpa* – a form that it is not, *pratiṣṭham* – established

1.9 *śabda* – word, *jñāna* – knowledge, *anupātī* – formed from, *vastu* – object, *śūnyaḥ* – empty, *vikalpaḥ* – imagination

1.10 *abhāva* – absence, *pratyaya* – subtle mind, *ālambanā* – support, *tamaḥ* – inertia, *vṛttir* – activities of the mind, *nidrā* – deep sleep

1.11 *anubhūta* – born from experience, *viṣaya* – object, *asaṁpramoṣaḥ* – never dies, *smṛtiḥ* – memory

1.12 *abhyāsa* – through practice, *vairāgyābhyāṁ* – by means of non-attachment, *tan* – of these, *nirodhaḥ* – ability to envelop

1.13 *tatra* – here, *sthitau* – to stay, *yatnaḥ* – effort, *abhyāsaḥ* – practice

1.14 *sa* – that, *tu* – indeed, *dīrgha* – long, *kāla* – time, *nairantarya* – without break, *satkāra* – positive attitude, *ādarā* – eagerness, *āsevitaḥ* – endowed with, *dṛḍha* – firm, *bhūmiḥ* – foundation

1.15 *dṛṣṭa* – perceptible, *ānuśravika* – heard, *viṣaya* – objects, *vitṛṣṇasya* – lack of desire, *vaśīkāra* – mastery, *saṁjñā* – known, *vairāgyam* – non-attachment

1.16 *tat* – that, *paraṁ* – ultimate, *puruṣa* – conscious principle, *khyāteḥ* – is known, *guṇa* – constituent qualities of nature, *vaitṛṣṇyam* – no thirst due to

1.17 *vitarka* – gross reflection, *vicāra* – subtle reflection, *ānanda* – beatitude, *asmitā* – being conscious of oneself, *rūpa* – form, *anugamāt* – following, *saṁprajñātaḥ* – total understanding

1.18 *virāma* – cessation, *pratyaya* – subtle mind, *abhyāsa* – practice, *pūrvaḥ* – preceded by, *saṁskāra* – behavioural patterns, *śeṣaḥ* – sleeping, *anyaḥ* – other

1.19 *bhava* – state of being, *pratyayaḥ* – special mind, *videha* – special body, *prakṛtilayānām* – those sensitive to nature

1.20 *śraddhā* – belief, *vīrya* – inner strength, *smṛti* – memory, *samādhi* – integration, *prajñā* – highest knowledge, *pūrvaka* – the previous, *itareṣām* – others

1.21 *tīvra* – intense, *saṁvegānām* – through great speed, *āsannaḥ* – near

1.22 *mṛdu* – gentle, *madhya* – moderate, *adhimātratvāt* – intense, *tataḥ* – then, *api* – also, *viśeṣaḥ* – specific differences

1.23 *īśvara* – source of light, *praṇidhānāt* – completely, continuously hold, *vā* – or/only

1.24 *kleśa* – cause of suffering, *karma* – actions, *vipāka* – consequences, *āśayaiḥ* – impressions, *aparāmṛṣṭaḥ* – untouched, *puruṣa* – conscious principle, *viśeṣa* – special, *īśvaraḥ* – source of light

1.25 *tatra* – in that, *niratiśayaṁ* – unlimited, *sarva* – all, *jña* – knowledge, *bījam* – seed

1.26 *saḥ* – it, *eṣaḥ* – indeed, *pūrveṣām* – preceding, *api* – even, *guruḥ* – teachers, *kālena* – through time, *anavacchedāt* – uninterrupted

1.27 *tasya* – of it, *vācakaḥ* – speak, *praṇavaḥ* – sacred sound

1.28 *tad* – of this, *japaḥ* – repetition, *tad* – its, *artha* – essence, *bhāvanam* – visualize

1.29 *tataḥ* – then, *pratyak* – inner, *cetanā* – consciousness, *adhigamaḥ* – attainment, *api* – also, *antarāya* – obstacles, *abhāvaḥ* – reduction, *ca* – and

1.30 *vyādhi* – disease, *styāna* – mental dullness, *saṁśaya* – doubt, *pramāda* – hastiness, *ālasya* – apathy, *avirati* – excessive sensual activity, *bhrāntidarśana* – distorted self-perception, *alabdhabhūmikatva* – inability to persevere, *anavasthitatvāni* – regression, *citta* – mind, *vikṣepāḥ* – distracted, *te* – these, *antarāyāḥ* – obstacles

1.31 *duḥkha* – emotional suffering, *daurmanasya* – negative thinking, *aṅgamejayatva* – agitated physiology, *śvāsa praśvāsāḥ* – disturbed breathing, *vikṣepa* – fickle mind, *saha bhuvaḥ* – accompanies

1.32 *tat* – that, *pratiṣedha* – to counter, *artham* – purpose, *eka* – one, *tattva* – essential principle, *abhyāsaḥ* – practise

1.33 *maitrī* – friendship, *karuṇā* – compassion, *mudita* – appreciated, *upekṣāṇāṁ* – equanimity, *sukha* – joyful, *duḥkha* – suffering, *puṇya* – virtue, *apuṇya* – vice, *viṣayāṇāṃ* – focus, *bhāvanātaḥ* – attitude, *citta* – mind, *prasādanam* – peaceful

1.34 *pracchardana* – exhaling, *vidhāraṇābhyāṁ* – retention, *vā* – or, *prāṅasya* – of the breath

1.35 *viṣayavatī* – objective perception, *vā* – or, *pravṛttiḥ* – development, *utpannā* – source, *manasaḥ* – of the mind, *sthiti* – steadiness, *nibandhinī* – achieved

1.36 *viśokā* – absence of pain, *vā* – or, *jyotiṣmatī* – full of light

1.37 *vīta* – devoid, *rāga* – desire, *viṣayaṃ* – object, *vā* – or, *cittam* – mind

1.38 *svapna* – dreams, *nidrā* – sleep, *jñāna* – knowledge, *ālambanaṁ* – support, *vā* – or

1.39 *yathā* – as is, *abhimata* – appropriate, *dhyānāt* – meditation, *vā* – or

1.40 *paramāṇu* – infinitely subtle, *parama* – supreme, *mahattva* – vastness, *antaḥ* – limit, *asya* – in its, *vaśīkāraḥ* – mastery over

1.41 *kṣīṇa* – reduced, *vṛtteḥ* – activities, *abhijātasya* – sparkles, *eva* – as if, *maṇeḥ* – jewels, *grahītṛ* – that which perceives, *grahaṇa* – that which does the perceiving, *grāhyeṣu* – that which is perceived, *tat stha* – in that state, *tad* – its, *añjanatā* – radiant quality, *samāpattiḥ* – contemplative integration

1.42 *tatra* – there, *śabda* – hear, *artha* – meaning, *jñāna* – knowledge, *vikalpaiḥ* – imagination, *saṇkīrṇā* – contaminated, *savitarkā* – with gross, *samāpattiḥ* – contemplative integration

1.43 *smṛti* – memory, *pariśuddhau* – completely cleaned, *svarūpa* – its own nature, *śūnya* – disappears, *iva* – as if, *artha mātra nirbhāsā* – only the focus shines, *nirvitarkā* – without gross

1.44 *etayā eva* – similarly, *savicārā* – with subtle, *nirvicārā* – without subtle, *ca* – and, *sūkṣma* – subtle, *viṣayā* – object, *vyākhyātā* – are known

1.45 *sūkṣma* – subtle, *viṣayatvaṁ* – being an object, *ca* – and, *aliṅga* – unmanifest, *paryavasānam* – reaches final stage

1.46 *tāḥ* – they, *eva* – indeed, *sabījaḥ* – with seed, *samādhiḥ* – integration

1.47 *nirvicāra* – without subtle, *vaiśāradye* – when mastered, *adhyātma* – the consciousness, *prasādaḥ* – is known

1.48 *ṛtaṁ* – highest truth, *bharā* – full of, *tatra* – there, *prajñā* – highest knowledge

1.49 *śrutā* – heard, *anumāna* – inferred, *prajñābhyām* – highest knowledge, *anya* – other, *viṣayā* – objects, *viśeṣa* – specific, *arthatvāt* – meaning

1.50 *tat* – this, *jaḥ* – born of, *saṁskāraḥ* – behavioural patterns, *anya* – other, *saṁskāra* – behavioural patterns, *pratibandhī* – replaces

1.51 *tasyaḥ* – that, *api* – even, *nirodhe* – enveloped state, *sarva* – all, *nirodhāt* – through absence of, *nirbījaḥ* – without seed, *samādhiḥ* – integration

iti – this, *prathama* – first, *samādhi* – integration, *pādaḥ* – chapter

Appendix II: Chapter Two of the Yoga Sūtra

atha – now, *sādhana* – practice, *pādaḥ* – chapter

2.1 *tapaḥ* – intense discipline, *svādhyāya* – reflective self-study, *īśvara praṇidhānāni* – accepting attitude / reverence, *kriyā yogaḥ* – yoga in action

2.2 *samādhi* – integration, *bhāvana* – feeling of, *arthaḥ* – purpose, *kleśa* – cause of suffering, *tanūkaraṇa* – reduced, *arthaḥ* – benefit, *ca* – and

2.3 *avidyā* – not knowing, *asmitā* – ego, *rāga* – desire, *dveṣa* – aversion, *abhiniveśāḥ* – fear, *kleśāḥ* – cause of suffering

2.4 *avidyā* – not knowing, *kṣetram* – the field, *uttareṣām* – for those who follow, *prasupta* – dormant, *tanu* – reduced, *vicchinna* – interrupted, *udārāṇām* – expanded

2.5 *anitya* – impermanent, *aśuci* – unclean, *duḥkha* – suffering, *anātmasu* – unconscious, *nitya* – permanent, *śuci* – clean, *sukha* – joy, *ātma* – conscious, *khyātiḥ* – knowing, *avidyā* – not knowing

2.6 *dṛg* – to see, *darśana* – perceived, *śaktyoḥ* – the power, *eka* – one, *ātmatā* – feeling of being, *iva* – as if, *asmitā* – ego / i-am-ness

2.7 *sukha* – joy, *anuśayī* – pursue, *rāgaḥ* – desire

2.8 *duḥkha* – emotional suffering, *anuśayī* – pursue, *dveṣaḥ* – aversion

2.9 *svarasa* – its own essence, *vāhī* – to flow, *viduṣaḥ* – for the wise, *api* – even, *samārūḍhaḥ* – deeply rooted, *abhiniveśaḥ* – fear

2.10 *te* – they, *pratiprasava* – impotent, *heyāḥ* – prevented, *sūkṣmāḥ* – subtle

2.11 *dhyāna* – through meditation, *heyāḥ* – prevented, *tad* – its, *vṛttayaḥ* – activities

2.12 *kleśa* – cause of suffering, *mūlaḥ* – source, *karma* – actions, *āśayaḥ* – impressions, *dṛṣṭa* – visible, *adṛṣṭa* – not visible, *janma* – born, *vedanīyaḥ* – experienced

2.13 *sati* – being, *mūle* – the root, *tad* – that, *vipākaḥ* – consequences, *jāti* – individual nature, *āyuḥ* – duration/time, *bhogāḥ* – the experience / the result

2.14 *te* – they, *hlāda* – joyful, *paritāpa* – repeated pain, *phalāḥ* – the fruits, *puṇya* – noble, *apuṇya* – ignoble, *hetutvāt* – the cause

2.15 *pariṇāma* – change, *tāpa* – deep thirst, *saṁskāra* – behavioural patterns, *duḥkhaiḥ* – emotional suffering, *guṇa* – inherent quality of matter, *vṛtti* – activities, *virodhāt* – imbalances, *ca* – and, *duḥkham* – emotional suffering, *eva* – even, *sarvaṁ* – everything, *vivekinaḥ* – for the wise

2.16 *heyaṁ* – prevent, *duḥkham* – emotional suffering, *anāgatam* – future

2.17 *draṣṭṛ* – the perceiver, *dṛśyayoḥ* – the perceived, *saṁyogo* – intense link, *heya* – symptoms, *hetuḥ* – cause

2.18 *prakāśa* – illuminate, *kriyā* – action, *sthiti* – structure, *īlaṁ* – qualities, *bhūta* – elements, *indriya* – sense organs, *ātmakaṁ* – constituent nature, *bhoga* – enjoyment, *apavarga* – freedom, *arthaṁ* – purpose, *dṛśyam* – the perceived

2.19 *viśeṣa* – the specific, *aviśeṣa* – the non-specific, *liṅgamātra* – potent only, *aliṅgāni* – impotent, *guṇa* – inherent quality of matter, *parvāṇi* – states

2.20 *draṣṭā* – the perceiver, *dṛśi* – perception, *mātraḥ* – only, *śuddhaḥ* – clean, *api* – even though, *pratyaya* – through subtle mind, *anupaśyaḥ* – perceives

2.21 *tad* – that, *artha* – purpose, *eva* – only, *dṛśyasya* – the perceived, *ātmā* – nature

2.22 *kṛtārthaṁ* – purpose fulfilled, *prati* – in respect of, *naṣṭam* – lost, *api* – yet, *anaṣṭaṁ* – not lost, *tad* – it, *anya* – for another, *sādhāraṇatvāt* – by becoming not owned

2.23 *sva* – itself in form, *svāmi* – the master, *śaktyoḥ* – power of, *svarūpa* – their own nature, *upalabdhi* – to obtain, *hetuḥ* – cause, *saṁyogaḥ* – intense link

2.24 *tasya* – its, *hetuḥ* – cause, *avidyā* – not knowing

2.25 *tad* – that, *abhāvāt* – through reduction, *saṁyogāḥ* – intense link, *abhāvo* – reduced, *hānaṁ* – goal, *tad* – that, *dṛśeḥ* – the perceiver, *kaivalyam* – freedom

2.26 *viveka khyātiḥ* – discriminative wisdom, *aviplavā* – unlimited, *hāna* – goal, *upāyaḥ* – near

2.27 *tasya* – of it, *saptadhā* – seven, *prānta* – distinct, *bhūmiḥ* – levels, *prajñā* – knowledge

2.28 *yoga* – yoga, *āṅga* – limbs, *anuṣṭhānāt* – practice, *aśuddhi* – impurities, *kṣaye* – remove, *jñāna* – knowledge, *dīptiḥ* – to light, *āviveka* – discernment / limitless clarity in action, *khyāteḥ* – in recognizing

2.29 *yama* – social attitudes, *niyama* – personal attitudes, *āsana* – posture, *prāṇāyāma* – regulation of breath, *pratyāhāra* – mastery of senses, *dhāraṇā* – capacity to focus, *dhyāna* – meditation, *samādhayaḥ* – integration, *aṣṭau* – eight, *aṅgāni* – limbs

2.30 *ahiṁsā* – non-violence, *satya* – truth, *asteya* – non-stealing, *brahmacarya* – appropriate relationships, *aparigrahāḥ* – non-grasping, *yamāḥ* – social attitudes

2.31 *jāti* – role, *deśa* – place, *kāla* – time, *samaya* – circumstance, *anavacchinnāḥ* – not interrupted, *sārva bhaumāḥ* – all levels, *mahā* – the great, *vratam* – commitment

2.32 *śauca* – cleanliness, *santoṣa* – contentment, *tapaḥ* – intense discipline, *svādhyāya* – self-reflection, *īśvara praṇidhānāni* – attitude of acceptance, *niyamāḥ* – personal attitudes

2.33 *vitarka* – hurtful actions, *bādhane* – to prevent, *pratipakṣa* – another perspective, *bhāvanam* – visualize

2.34 *vitarkāḥ* – gross actions, *hiṁsa* – violence, *ādayaḥ* – etc., *kṛta* – do it oneself, *kārita* – get it done, *anumoditāḥ* – someone else does it, *lobha* – greed, *krodha* – anger, *moha* – deluded, *pūrvakāḥ* – due to, *mṛdu* – gentle, *madhya* – medium, *adhimātrāḥ* – intense, *duḥkha* – suffering, *ajñāna* – lack of clarity, *ananta* – endless, *phalāḥ* – fruits, *iti* – therefore, *pratipakṣa* – different perspective, *bhāvanam* – visualize

2.35 *ahiṁsā* – non-violence, *pratiṣṭhāyāṁ* – firmly established in, *tat* – this, *sannidhau* – near presence, *vaira* – animosity, *tyāgaḥ* – abandoned

2.36 *satya* – truth, *pratiṣṭhāyāṁ* – firmly established in, *kriyā* – action, *phala* – fruits of, *śrayatvam* – well supported

2.37 *asteya* – non-stealing, *pratiṣṭhāyāṁ* – firmly established in, *sarva* – all, *ratna* – jewels, *upasthānam* – stay near

2.38 *brahmacarya* – appropriate relationships, *pratiṣṭhāyāṁ* – firmly established in, *vīrya* – inner strength, *lābhaḥ* – obtained

2.39 *aparigraha* – non-grasping, *sthairye* – being steady in, *janma* – birth, *kathaṁtā* – the reason of, *saṁbodhaḥ* – total knowledge

2.40 *śaucāt* – through cleanliness, *svāṅga* – one's own body parts, *jugupsā* – disgust, *paraiḥ* – others, *asaṁsargaḥ* – disconnect

2.41 *sattva* – clear mind, *śuddhi* – cleaning, *saumanasya* – positive thinking, *aikāgrya* – focusing, *indriya* – sense organs, *jaya* – mastered, *ātma* – inner being, *darśana* – vision, *yogyatvāni* – attitude for, *ca* – and

2.42 *santoṣāt* – through contentment, *anuttamaḥ* – the highest, *sukha* – joy, *lābhaḥ* – gained

2.43 *kāya* – body, *indriya* – senses, *siddhiḥ* – mastery of, *aśuddhi* – of the unclean, *kṣayāt* – through reduction, *tapasaḥ* – intense discipline

2.44 *svādhyāyāt* – through self-reflection, *iṣṭa* – desired, *devatā* – deity, *samprayogaḥ* – deep connection

2.45 *samādhi* – integration, *siddhiḥ* – mastery, *īśvara praṇidhānāt* – accepting attitude

2.46 *sthira* – stable, *sukham* – comfortable, *āsanam* – posture

2.47 *prayatna* – appropriate effort, *śaithilya* – loosening, *ananta* – endless, *samāpattibhyām* – through meditation

2.48 *tataḥ* – then, *dvandvān* – the opposites, *abhighātaḥ* – not affected

2.49 *tasmin* – in that, *sati* – established, *śvāsa* – inhaling, *praśvāsayoḥ* – exhaling, *gati* – movement, *vicchedaḥ* – to cut, *prāṇāyāmaḥ* – regulated breathing

2.50 *āhya* – exhale, *ābhyantara* – inhale, *stambha* – retention, *vṛttiḥ* – activity, *deśa* – place, *kāla* – time, *saṁkhyābhiḥ* – number, *paridṛṣṭo* – carefully observed, *dīrgha* – long, *sūkṣmaḥ* – smooth

2.51 *bāhya* – external, *ābhyantara* – internal, *viṣaya* – object, *ākṣepī* – transcend, *caturthaḥ* – the fourth

2.52 *tataḥ* – then, *kṣīyate* – removed, *prakāśa* – the light, *āvaraṇam* – surrounding veil

2.53 *dhāraṇāsu* – for concentration, *ca* – and, *yogyatā* – becomes ready, *manasaḥ* – the mind

2.54 *svaviṣaya* – its own object, *asaṁprayoge* – distinct from, *cittasya* – of mind, *svarūpa* – its own, *anukāraḥ* – to follow, *iva* – as if, *indriyāṇāṁ* – the senses, *pratyāhāraḥ* – opposite food

2.55 *tataḥ* – as a consequence, *paramā* – highest, *vaśyatā* – mastery, *indriyāṇāṁ* – the senses

iti – this, *dvitīyaḥ* – second, *sādhana* – practice, *pādaḥ* – chapter

Further Reading

Desikachar, T. K. V., *The Heart of Yoga: Developing a Personal Practice* (Inner Traditions, 1999)

Mohan, A. G. and Indra Mohan *Yoga Therapy: A Guide to the Therapeutic Use of Yoga and Ayurveda for Health and Fitness* (Shambhala Publications Inc., 2004)

Mohan, A. G., *Krishnamacharya: His Life and Teachings* (Shambhala Publications Inc., 2010)

Bouanchaud, B., *Meditation: Techniques in the Yoga Tradition* (London, Deśa Publishing, 2019)

Cope, Stephen, *Yoga and the Quest for the True Self* (Bantam Books Inc., 2000)

Nestor, James, *Breath: The New Science of a Lost Art* (Penguin Life, 2021)

True Yoga: www.TrueYoga.co.uk

British Council of Yoga Therapy: www.bcyt.org

International Association of Yoga Therapists: www.iayt.org

Acknowledgements

Thank you to Venetia at Penguin for believing in me and commissioning this book. Then to Emily, Anya and the rest of the team at Penguin who took it to where it is now. To Helen, who worked with me online day after day through multiple Covid lockdowns, asked all the right questions, stress-tested yoga philosophy to an extreme and brought this book to life. You were amazing to work with – thank you. I'm grateful to each of the clients I have worked with over the last twenty years: a sincerest thank you to you all. To Miranda, Saffron and Freddie, thank you for your unconditional love and support.